MY MEDICINE, MY BODY

Basil Porter

To Ron & Di —

In love &
friendship — despite
the distance.

Basil
June 2017

MY MEDICINE, MY BODY

The Serious Physician becomes a Serious Patient

Basil Porter

To Noga, Keren, Dana, and Ron -
for being there when I needed you

To Ruth Avram and Mark Clarfeld
for egging me on and providing good advice

To Daniella -
for much patience and guidance
as well as editing skill

KIP – Kotarim International Publishing, Ltd.

Edited by: Daniella Maor
Graphic Design by: Bat-Chen Nachmani

Publisher: Moshe Alon

ISBN: 978-965-7589-19-9
Printed in Israel 2016

"No one else sees the world the way you do, so no one else can tell the stories that you have to tell."

Charles de Lint, writer (b. 22 Dec 1951)

CONTENTS

INTRODUCTION

As I have moved along my career pathway in medicine I have had a dream, surely shared by hundreds of other physicians, that my personal story might be something special enough to interest other people. Did I have the ability of the brilliant Harvard surgeon Atul Guwande to write about medicine in a way that would appeal not only to a narrow group of specialists in a particular field, but also to a lay public interested in issues of their health?

I realised that the publishing houses would not be waiting for a book written by a paediatrician in Israel to share stories about child health or the problems facing health care systems. From time to time I would write a short article and try getting it published in one of the columns of the prestigious journals dedicated to personal stories and anecdotes, pieces not requiring rigid research data and statistical values. I was proud when an article I wrote about my lonely experience with a number of patients with death and near-death situations finally appeared in a Canadian journal. I thought of writing about studying and practicing medicine in South Africa, America, the UK, and Israel, to try and uncover the cultural and political differences which influence the personal experience of a physician in each of these countries, but realised that in this global village there are many physicians with far more interesting experiences.

And then, at the beginning of my seventh decade, and as I entered a period of retirement from active involvement in medicine, a series of serious personal experiences with my health took center stage. I suddenly saw my body as a story, a unique story with many lessons to be learnt. What my experience as a paediatrician, health services manager, and medical academician had not provided as substance for an interesting tale, was now offered by serendipity. As my series of bodily events spurred me to reflect on my personal existence and the state of the medical profession, I had become my own laboratory, needing only to look inwards and learn what these events had taught me.

Medical science focuses on the proven scientific

method. So when we say that a smallpox or measles vaccine prevents disease, the data prove it. This is not some opinion of a crank, but proof from years of painstaking study. Most of the learning about diagnosis and treatment of disease today is based on the facts of good science.

In my student days, fifty years ago, most of clinical medicine was based on wise doctors talking about "in my experience". Chromosomes had only recently been properly documented, and the lecture on the structure of DNA was about a new discovery. Our revered professor of surgery berated keyhole surgery, insisting that any decent surgeon needed to make an adequate wide incision in order to operate properly. In the early 1980's my gallbladder was removed leaving a long scar under my right rib cage, probably one of the last of its kind. A decade later keyhole surgery became the mainstay of surgery, and since then almost all procedures are conducted through "keyholes". Gallbladders, appendices, and ovaries are all whisked out through keyholes with the help of an endoscope enabling visualisation of the affected organ.

Today, a good doctor knows that when a patient swears that drinking a mixture of onion and honey every morning has kept him fit, his opinion should be respected because he believes it has helped him. But unless there has been a serious study comparing this treatment with others there is no real reason the doctor should suggest this to other patients. Another primary tool for any practitioner, - a key part of doctoring, is the narrative, or at least it was. With twentieth century's explosion of scientifically-based cures for all man's ailments, including the use of computers for documentation, the narrative has shrunk. Young interns ask sets of pre-determined questions and enter them into the computer, using unintelligible abbreviations, and then send the patient for blood tests, or front-line imaging which should provide the diagnosis. If the patient tries to expand his story the doctor will hasten to return to the protocol, not wishing to be confused with further irrelevant feelings or complaints. The patient's story has been replaced by pointed questions, the stethoscope has given way to the echocardiogram, and the ultrasound and MRI machines have made the palpating hand a rarity. Have we forgotten the crucial importance of the physician as an agent for diagnosing and caring via careful listening and systematic clinical examination?

And so, I arrived at my idea to document my body as the object of study, and to try and learn lessons from a lifetime of experiences with different health problems. Could I borrow the transactional model commonly used in the field of child development, and use my personal experience with a health problem to learn how the system sets out to deal with it? The Transactional Model of Child Development suggests that along life's course there is a constant process of the environment influencing the child, as well as the child influencing the environment.

A depressed mother influences the behavior of her premature baby, while the premature baby is causing the mother's depression. Does the patient influence the health care environment? Does the doctor order more tests for a chronic hypochondriac patient? Will the obstetrician decide on a caesarian section more rapidly with a mother who is a lawyer concerned about having an abnormal baby? Did every doctor who had seen me during my disease episodes behave differently because I was a doctor? Did the fact I was a doctor affect my behavior as a patient? And to make things just a fraction more complicated, it's not just about the doctor and patient alone. This equation includes another intervening force - the health care system - affecting and maybe even determining the direction and nature of the encounter.

Commenting on the health care system requires a peek into the state of medical care, or the "state of health of the population" as my teacher the late Sydney Kark would prefer to say. We look at the obvious: how long do people live in the country, how many infants die in the first year of life, and how many women die during childbirth? I don't know what the figures were back then in apartheid South Africa, the land of my birth, but certainly the white population was among the top in the world, while among the blacks it was third world levels. Today in Israel where I live, life expectancy is among the highest in the world, infant mortality is among the lowest in the western world, and a death in childbirth is a rarity. So things are pretty good compared with Somalia. But if you go and ask people about experience with health and disease, most will probably have some misery stories about the process of getting health care. These stories do not appear in the country's health ratings - a trendy idea in medicine that has recently become popular. Why the number of heart catheterisations performed in one state of the USA is double compared to the adjacent state? Why nearly a third of labours in a particular country end in a caesarian section? Why are the people of Japan much healthier than Americans, yet spending less than a half of what Americans spend on health care? These questions, and their answers, along with other facts and figures contribute to the understanding of the state of health of the population. But in the long run what counts is the result for the patient. Not just whether he or she are alive after a medical experience or procedure, but how did it affect them?

A doctor who writes about his own experience with disease and health systems faces a special challenge. Any description of symptoms or aspects of his problems will be coloured and probably distorted by his knowledge and experience, and certainly by his probable denial of symptoms. A doctor can never stop being the doctor, trying to reason and explain as a medical scientist, while experiencing subjective aches, pains, and morbid thoughts that any patient with a new disease will feel. Frequently the doctor might not be honest with himself, using denial or cynicism to justify lack of action. In addition, the environment will have different expectations from the sick physician. Family will assume the doctor knows how to look after himself, and his colleagues will assume he knows what to do. The sick physician is the classic cobbler who walks barefoot. This unique experience, being a physician and experiencing my maladies, has enabled me to reflect on the interface between the patient and the health care system from both perspectives, and so my stories touch on a spectrum of topical issues in medicine such as acute care, emergency care, developing medical technology, cutting-edge cancer diagnosis and treatment, the role of super-specialists, and catastrophic care.

Looking back, I realise that in some cases cure was unquestionably related to the amazing advances in medicine during my lifetime, while other problems resolved despite, not because of the medical system. While at least some credit to recovery should be granted to my genes, I would also like to believe that changes I had made in my lifestyle had contributed to the end result as well. Why and how did I stop smoking? How did I get hooked onto jogging? Have I really tried to manipulate a healthier eating style for myself? Has yoga helped me to be healthier in mind and body? Has a forty-one year marriage, with three children and five grandchildren living in relative harmony with each other, helped prevent depression and heart attacks? Has a passion for playing chamber music been an enabler of inner peace and better ability to deal with adversity? And how much has just been luck, or a guiding hand from above, according to one's beliefs?

The personal experience of disease, pain, and suffering is insulting to the doctor. The doctor as the patient has a lonely role. He is expected to not feel the doubts and concerns regarding his condition, to tolerate the symptoms better, to be a braver warrior facing the forces waging against his health. Sadly, the opposite is probably true. He will often have some knowledge of the condition, through memories of a lecture or a patient in medical school, but he will not be fully up-to-date on a condition not within his field of expertise. In the words of the old proverb, the little knowledge becomes a dangerous thing.

When I received the diagnosis of a tumour of the parotid gland requiring head and neck surgery, my mind immediately flashed back to my medical school lectures. Head and neck surgery meant putting a tube in the trachea[1] to enable the patient to breathe, being fed through a stomach tube, almost always resulting in deformity due to damage to nerves. I lived with these thoughts for two weeks while waiting for my surgery, only to be told by the surgeon that things were not done that way anymore, and nerve injury was relatively rare in the procedure I would undergo. As doctors we will minimise or maximise symptoms and their significance, and objectivity proves to be almost

---

1. Also called the windpipe. The tube allowing the passage of air from the throat down to the lungs.

impossible to achieve. We are denied the luxury of ignorance, while living with the unreliability of limited knowledge.

This had led me to the thought that what we need is probably a niche sub-specialty called "a doctors' doctor". A special track whereby doctors learn about the unique difficulties of being a doctor-patient, and the special needs involved. As I realise this is unlikely to come about, I can take some comfort and offer some reassurance that some of these animals do exist. They have not undergone a specific specialty certification, but have mastered their art and taught themselves to approach patients with the right disposition no matter if they are laymen or doctors. These special breeds of doctors use their knowledge and skills to care for scared doctors who have found themselves thrust into the patient role. They are able to radiate their high-level professional expertise together with the basic skills of empathy, showing the concerned doctor-patient that they are in control of the situation, and understand how this particular doctor-patient feels.

I think that being a patient through a range of experiences has been humbling, to say the least. At the most basic and most important level, each has been a reminder that it could, and in fact did, happen. The other piece to this is the fact that life depends not so much on what hand you are dealt, but rather what you do with it. In my case, playing the hand depended on the state of medical science and technology, the people using them - the good surgeon or physician, and the coping - probably related to how I dealt with it all, via my character or inherent resilience.

So while my story trumpets the triumphs of medical technology achievements in saving lives and alleviating suffering, I also have been aware of the many moments when the system has failed to care for me. My personal journey through the pathology book has heightened my awareness regarding the need for both a sympathetic ear and an expert caring hand. The narrative that emerges from my series of bodily trials is meant to try and highlight both for me and for my readers the complex processes of ill-health and medical care. My stories through my memory are aimed to try and focus on the process of the initial breakdown of the healthy organ, through the personal experience of symptoms, the diagnostic process, and the therapeutic pathway. I believe that in the final analysis of medical care we will always need to try and follow this pathway, learning the necessary lessons from science and the particular human being with a certain disease. Perhaps this is the true meaning of comprehensive care. I have read numerous books about how doctors see the process of health care and have learnt a lot from them, but there is something unique about the opportunity that fate has thrown my way - a baggage of diagnoses affecting almost every organ or system in my body and yet seemingly allowing me to carry on functioning.

Last but not least, while writing my story, I realised there was another issue I faced - the fickleness of memory. At a time when I find myself cursing at least three times a day that I cannot remember a name of a person, place, book, or piece of music, how can I possibly expect to remember details of an illness twenty, thirty, or fifty years ago? I can only hope that the parts remembered clearly, requiring some conscious or unconscious improvisation, compensate for the vaguer parts.

In the subsequent chapters I will present my experience with my body enduring a number of problems; some unpleasant but rather common and relatively benign, while others indeed serious and life-threatening. I have found myself to be a "natural experiment", an example of one person looking at himself from two perspectives. A person trying to reflect on the many occasions he has had to test his body and the system, while he happens to be a medical man. Hopefully, my thoughts and conclusions will help other potential patients and their doctors to understand a little better the complexity of health care today - the incredible challenges catalyzed by rapid technological advancements, alongside the slow seeming dissipation of humanism and compassion.

THE SOREST TUMMY

I was twelve years old, and was already showing signs of a paediatric future. I adored little kids, and when my parents befriended a couple much younger than them with a one-year-old son, my greatest joy was being able to babysit. Not just watch him sleep for a couple of hours while his parents were out to dinner, but spend a full day playing with him in the playground, in his playroom, and feeding him at mealtimes. I admit this was a bit strange for an early teenager to prefer the company of a toddler to a movie with his peers, but looking back, this early fascination with babies was probably an important step in my later career pathway.

It was a Sunday afternoon, and the family of my

baby friend had invited me to join them on a trip to the local drive-in café, famous for its milkshakes and toasted sandwiches. I remember well having my usual toasted cheese and strawberry milkshake, and then being taken back home. At this point, I was aware of what we would call a tummy ache, nothing very unusual. Traveling in my memory over fifty years back, the scene is still very vivid. I was alone at home, amusing myself in my room, and slowly the ache increased. Two hours later there was no question that this pain was something new. It was not fading away as the usual tummy ache did, but rather increasing in steady waves, till I was rolling around on my bed. By the time my parents returned, they took one look at me and realised that this was indeed something extraordinary. My mother, who did not usually show the behavioral pattern of the typical Jewish mother, immediately suggested I eat something, and despite my explanation of the milkshake and sandwich a few hours earlier, minutes later I was being coaxed to swallow some scrambled eggs on toast, my favorite Sunday night meal. This would prove to be a very relevant event regarding the subsequent unfolding of the surgical saga.

And so, even though it was ten pm on a Sunday night, Dr. C our family general practitioner was called. After taking a brief look at me, he understood pretty quickly that this was something more serious than the usual "tummy upset". Also, this time his examination included something new from the routine I knew, as he placed a rubber glove over his hand and explained to me that he was going to put his finger in my bum, and it would be a little unpleasant. As I remember, the stomach pains were so bad at this point that had he said he was going to amputate my leg, I would not have responded. So the rectal examination was completed, and Dr C's face looked even more serious than before. By the time he was through with his examination it was eleven pm. Yet, the laboratory was called and the technician arrived to take blood for a blood count and a urine specimen. The laboratory results arrived around midnight, and at this point Dr C told my very worried parents that he wanted a surgical opinion.

It was already around one o'clock on Monday morning when Mr M the surgeon arrived. The only thing I remember was that he looked quite old to me and did not smile. Again he asked all the questions and examined my stomach. Then with a very serious look, he took my parents aside and said that he had to operate. At around two o'clock in the morning I was bundled in a coat and driven to the nursing home, the private hospital where the surgery would be performed. I remember clearly that I was wide awake and aware at this time, and I think the pains had subsided a little. Because when my father stopped the car in the deserted hospital car park next to a sign "For Doctors Only", I told him that this was not permissible. He smiled and assured me it was all right. As my father was a very law abiding lawyer, I guessed this was OK.

At around three am on a Monday morning, I found myself lying on a trolley looking up at the bright lights of the operating room, with lots of people fussing around. I remember someone explaining that I was going to have a mask on my face, and then the darkness, the amazing visit to nothingness that little did I know I would experience a few more times during my life journey. I think this first anaesthetic experience had a major effect on my thoughts about death. As a kid, I thought a lot about death, not because of any particularly traumatic experiences, but just as something that I thought should concern me. The main thing that worried me about dying was the idea that you left the earthly experience, and that no one really knew what happened afterwards. To me, the scary part of death was the idea that I would leave this earth and still be able to see what was going on, but not be involved. The loneliness in this idea scared me, and then came this anaesthetic experience which suggested that there was no loneliness, there was basically, well, nothing. A heavy thought for a twelve-year-old boy.

While I was in the heavy darkness, there was lots of action going on in the operating room. Here, I have to rely on my parents stories, relayed by Dr C, who assisted the surgeon in the operating room. It seems that the surgeon had performed what is known as an explorative laparotomy[2], basically meaning that he did not know what was going on in my stomach and would therefore have

2. A surgical procedure involving a large incision through the abdominal wall to gain access into the abdominal cavity

to "explore" my abdominal cavity in order to arrive at a diagnosis. So he made a long incision in the lower right part of the abdomen. At this stage, and while the surgeon and his team were hard at work with my open abdomen my toasted cheese, milkshake, and scrambled eggs began to exit from my stomach via my mouth. One does not have to be a trained medical person to understand that this is not a good thing to happen while someone is cutting open your tummy and you have a breathing tube down your throat. The vomiting was copious and life threatening and prolonged the surgery. Finally, the diagnosis was made, and an acutely inflamed appendix was removed and put in a bottle with formalin, and then placed next to my bed, so that the first thing I saw as I opened my eyes in the ward was a brown bottle with a yellowish worm like object floating in liquid.

I remember very clearly waking from the blackness to the voice of a nurse sitting next to my bed, telling me not to move around too much and that everything was fine. I eagerly asked if I could see the scar on my tummy before showing it to my friends, and remember the disappointment at finding only mounds of sticking plaster covering my stomach. The hospitalisation was long, a few weeks, with prolonged fevers causing lots of concern. I do remember that I felt pretty good most of the time, enjoying the attention and the gifts that streamed in with every visitor. I also fell in love with at least two of the young nurses looking after me, wondering whether there was a real possibility of having a relationship with them as soon as I was fully vertical again. And then there were another six weeks at home, carefully supervised by Dr C, with strict rules for rest, food and activity, my mother a faithful and willing accomplice to any decision of his. Finally, the plaster had been removed to reveal a very long cut alongside my belly button, a rather ugly wormy looking addition to my abdominal area, its lack of aesthetics easily balanced in my eyes by the sympathy it induced in the environment.

Looking back on this major experience as a doctor, there are quite a few lessons to be learnt. Firstly, it was clear that something was really wrong when the stomach aches lasted so long with such increasing severity. I don't think that one had to be a brilliant diagnostician to know that this was not a run of the mill "upset tummy", as it was called in local Lower Houghton lingo. Secondly, there is a clear reason for a doctor to ask a patient (or his mother) when did he eat or drink, the moment a suspicion arises that urgent surgery might be necessary. Strawberry milkshake plus scrambled eggs on toast do not go well with anaesthetics and knives opening the abdominal cavity. I think I will not be exaggerating if I say that there was serious concern for my survival as I threw up all over the operating room during surgery. Thirdly, this episode happened just before the realization that contrary to accepted practice, one must get the post-operative patient moving as soon as possible after the surgery, usually the following morning, and not leave him lying around in bed for a few weeks without moving.

So how would the whole story look like if happening fifty years later? I have never been too close to operating rooms (or theaters as they were known in the British Empire where I grew up), but from following developments in the area over the years, I can guess the following scenario. As soon as the stomach aches suggested something serious going on inside, probably the first test would be an ultrasound examination which would almost certainly have shown the fat, abnormal appendix and enabled a speedy decision regarding surgery. And the big change would be the type of surgery. The surgeon would make two little holes in the abdominal wall, insert a laparoscope, visualize the inflamed organ and remove it through one of the holes, or in worst-case scenario make a cut near the problem and remove it. The anaesthetic would be much more sophisticated, with less complications of vomiting, and the whole procedure would be over in an hour. The next morning I would be walking around the ward and I would be home within forty-eight hours. The scars would be two tiny slits where the laparoscope was used, and if further surgery had been necessary it would be a small scar on the right side. Also, I would not wake up with the appendix in a jar next to my bed. The appendix would be sent to a pathology laboratory for formal examination and confirmation of the diagnosis. But my mother would probably still force down some scrambled eggs.

Modern management of appendicitis has taken away much of the art, and yes, the fun of trying to make the clinical diagnosis accurate. Many hours of my medical student days were spent taking a history and examining the abdomen of a patient with suspected appendicitis. It was a classic test of clinical skill, whether on the medicine wards (to rule out the surgical diagnosis) or on the surgical wards (to verify the surgical diagnosis).There was little help from x-rays, and ultrasound was not yet an everyday clinical tool. It was also one of those tests of clinical diagnosis where there was a gold standard for knowing whether your diagnosis was correct, i.e. did the decision to operate show a "lily white", a normal appendix, or did it reveal the splendor of an inflamed appendix? The adage on the surgical wards was that the best surgeon had a score of seven out of ten, i.e. three out of ten operations were for a normal appendix. If you scored ten out of ten it was a sign that in your clinical life you were missing a few pathological appendices. There was no greater source of satisfaction as a student than to accompany the surgeon to surgery, see the inflamed appendix appear, and assist in its removal after having taken a history and examined a patient, declaring that this was appendicitis. Today, few medical students, even at the best medical schools, will have the opportunity to test and hone clinical skills as we did. Sophisticated laboratory tests and imaging procedures will be ordered after a minimal history and examination, and it is rare that a surgeon will stand next to a medical student, observing how he asks the patient the relevant questions and how he palpates the abdomen.

In my student days the ritual of assessing a child with a suspected acute abdomen was a key part of clinical training. No lecture, list of guidelines or algorithm could ever replace the clinical role models who showed me the right way to do this assessment. With warm hands, one started to gently palpate the stomach, all the time looking at the child's face to see if he was indicating increasing distress at any point. Then, pushing deeper into the stomach looking for the localisation of pain expected from the inflamed organ, while often having to distinguish between the child's crying that was due to the strange environment and unfamiliar faces, and his true cry from the inflamed appendix. This examination took time, and one usually sat down next to the patient to indicate that you intended to do a thorough job, using all the time required to get the correct picture.

Today, the results of the ultrasound or even the CAT scan of the abdomen will be presented to the attending surgeon, the clinical assessment of the acute abdomen a remnant of the past when medical diagnosis was dependent on the ears and the hands, without the help and dangers of modern technology. As a resident and then as a paediatrician, there were many opportunities to deal with the problem of stomach aches in children. My personal voyage with appendicitis was always there to remind me about the difference between an innocent, common tummy ache and the acute abdomen I had experienced. The skilled physician will always be the one who picks up the chart of the patient with the common complaint of abdominal pains, and know how to proceed through a careful history, which will almost invariably tell him if this is a benign or potentially serious problem, before shunting the child off to the laboratory or hospital. Children usually do not lie, and if they look sick, they often are truly sick. I think that even at the age of twelve I realised that I had a serious problem, long before the surgeon arrived. So as a young resident when I would push open the curtain to see the child with the stomach ache, I was always asking myself "Does he feel like I did that night?"

My appendicitis was my first serious illness. It was my first lesson in being truly in touch with my body, a first realization that something could go seriously wrong. This was a first experience of pain that was not transient, pain that dragged me down and stopped all ability to function normally. This was my first experience of a health problem that could not be solved in my own bed with the help of Dr C's house call. This was my first encounter with the wonders of a drug that would allow you to sleep while somebody took a sharp knife and cut open your abdomen. This was also my first lucky break, an encounter with a medical problem that could have proceeded to an early end to my life. With this, or any subsequent medical problem, there would always be the possibility of being saved by medical advances, while complications related to the disease or to mistakes in management, like knowing that one never operates on an abdomen when the stomach is still busy digesting a strawberry milkshake, toasted cheese sandwich and scrambled eggs, could easily change the result drastically.

ACNE MOST VULGAR

I don't remember exactly when it started, but at some stage I observed new hair growing in strange places on my body and experienced an unbelievable desire to sleep with Audrey Hepburn. Then, some small yellow bumps appeared on my face. From there things moved quickly, and by age fourteen my face and back were covered with pimples, zits or in professional terminology, *Acne vulgaris*.

I could deal with the pimples. They were quite predictable, a small yellow or black dot which over a few days developed into a bright yellow pustule. I learnt quite quickly to pop these lesions myself, helping them to ripen with some heat application.

There were also the lotions, the clear one for cleaning, then the brownish one which remained on the skin as a powdery haze, disguising the acne lesions but other than that not doing much, while the process moved inexorably onward as huge red cysts accompanied the blackheads and pustules. These had the habit of appearing on the side of the nose, then increasing in size causing the whole cheek to distend, and were always at their worst on the day I was due to date a new young lady. This was the stage when antibiotic creams, then pills were added to the regime.

I would look in the mirror realizing that there was no way that the prospective date would not notice. I saw what she would see - a face covered with yellow and black spots, a large red cyst on the side of the nose and numerous scars over the chin and forehead reflecting the graveyards of previous lesions. Not a handsome sight. The morning ablution became prolonged and complicated. First, there was the shaving, trying not to nick the lesions or prick open the cysts, followed by the acne therapeutic regime that began with the special soaps, followed by the cleansers, and then the drying agents and antibiotics.

At this fairly early stage of adolescent hormonal chaos I was referred to the local "skin chap" as my mother called him. Dr L was a Dickensian prototype; short, with wavy hair, horn-rimmed glasses and little chit-chat, certainly with the adolescent acne types. It was, "Hullo Basil", then straight to the examining couch. A little staring and prodding of the various lesions, then on to the prescriptions for the various bottles of lotions, mixtures, creams and ointments, always with the initial optimism that these would magically give my face and torso a baby's bottom cum-peaches-and-cream complexion. Nevertheless, the small yellow zits, hordes of blackheads alongside them, and the angry red cysts, the ultimate victory of the acne vulgaris bacteria and their cronies, spread in increasing numbers over my body. The evening ritual of cleaning the skin with cotton balls soaked in alcohol followed by the brown powdery mixture did nothing except make larger areas of the skin look red and blotchy. The antibiotic lotions followed by antibiotic pills showed zero impact on the attacking forces. The next step was attacking the enemy directly, with Dr L directing me to the examination couch and then starting to squeeze the pustules and blackheads and gouging the cysts with a sharp needle-type instrument. It hurt, first physically and then emotionally, when I would board the bus home with a batch of small pieces of adhesive plaster covering all the points of Dr L's attack. Only when I reached home and looked in the mirror did I realise that my fellow passengers had obviously considered the scenario suggestive of one of the great plague epidemics, and had respectfully kept their distance.

The visits to Dr L became a regular weekly routine, with no improvement noted. Dr L did not seem to be distressed by the lack of progress, changing the prescription for a lotion or antibiotic regularly and humming quietly as he jabbed the lesions before sending me on my way. When I expressed concern that after one year of treatment the disease process seemed totally untouched by the treatment, he obligingly suggested to my mother that I undergo a course of radiation therapy to the face. This was the era before demands for full disclosure and informed consent for everything done between physician and patient. Doctors were kings, and the default assumption was that anything the doctor suggested was in the patient's best interest.

So if Dr L thought I should be radiated that was the decision. I was ready for anything. I would have agreed to stand ten meters away from a meltdown of a nuclear plant, anything to be able to see a normal face again in the mirror. So instead of the gouging (or was it in addition to?), I would lie down while a conical machine hummed some rays at my face. I would imagine the cellular structure of the pustules and cysts quietly disintegrating, allowing for new virgin cells to take their place, smooth clear skin looking back at me in the mirror within a few days. But that was not to be, as the red, yellow and black additions to my face continued unabated.

I don't think Dr L was aware of the impact acne vulgaris had on a fifteen-year-old adolescent's life. When I would finally pluck up the courage to phone a girl for a date, and if successful, the stress period began in earnest. Would the state of my skin, at least on the face, improve between Monday night (the setting of the date) and Saturday night? I would spring out of bed to the bathroom in the morning, begging the guiding hand in heaven to hold the enemy back, but sure enough, by Friday morning either a huge angry yellow or black pimple would appear on the tip of my nose, or two new huge ugly red cysts would occupy the territory between the ear and the nose, or the chin, or anywhere fresh unblemished skin still remained. Then the frantic washing and scrubbing with special brushes and soaps, hoping that in the period until the meeting on Saturday night it might at least fade (I learnt early that hoping for disappearance of lesions was asking too much). Of course, today one knows that the rubbing and scrubbing just aggravated the inflammatory process of acne, but hindsight is of little help.

The bad, angry red cysts also had an amazing predilection to appear in the most visible and most painful places imaginable. One of these was the groove running alongside the side of the nose. The groove would start to feel a little tender, followed by increasing swelling and redness, the entire anatomy of the nose becoming distorted as the progressive enlarging red, angry, painful volcano dominated the face. It was truly center stage and the first thing anybody, particularly a young lady, would see. I speedily learnt that the natural history of these acne cysts was a long process, with no hope of the monster disappearing within less than two or three weeks, and also that the hot compresses and Dr L's gouger did little to change the course.

The other chosen place of honor for a cyst or a furuncle was the tip of the nose. My natural nose was not a classic Roman model, but rather of the more bulbous, Jewish kind. It certainly did not need anything to increase its conspicuous tip. But many of these large furuncles would appear there, starting again with the telltale slight tenderness and redness and then slowly but relentlessly progressing to the red-based, yellowish blob. I learnt over the years to test the readiness of the lesions for personal intervention, i.e. squeezing, with expulsion of the pus. If done at the right moment, the result would be rewarding, with the lesion dissolving rapidly and the skin returning to its normal condition. But if there was an urgent need to try and improve the appearance of my face for the Saturday night date, premature attempts at squeezing would result in agonizing pain and a massive increase in the redness surrounding the blob.

There was also a plethora of theories regarding prevention and management of the condition. Chocolate and fried foods, two passions of any normal adolescent were to be excluded. Some would talk of the therapeutic effects of good lovemaking, which was a particularly painful suggestion when one was encountering consistent refusal for anything even distantly approaching the desired act. Stress was also probably correctly implicated, but this was also not very helpful at a time when high school or medical school examinations came one after another, and it was not at all obvious that the condition improved during vacation time.

Acne trauma was not limited to Saturday night dates. A high point took place during a Latin class at school. The teacher was a notorious character, who would say the most inappropriate things at the most inappropriate times, always thinking he was working for the best interests of the student. As I struggled to memorize a passage from Ovid on a hot summer afternoon, I felt the small figure of Mr K, who always paraded between the isles of desks while silent study was in progress, stopping next to my desk. This could mean that there was about to be a reprimand for the poor score on a previous test, or a question why I had not attended a cricket practice the previous afternoon under his supervision. But Mr K always managed to introduce the element of surprise. I felt his arm affectionately patting my shoulder and his proclaiming out loud, for all the class to hear, "Don't worry little Porter, just keep putting your face toward the sun, and I'm sure things will improve". There was a short pause before the entire class of thirty five adolescent boys broke out in roars of laughter, while Mr K smiled with delight at the camaraderie his comment had produced.

Following this incident, fellow students would pass me on the playground with huge smiles repeating the mantra, "Don't worry little Porter, just keep your face in the sun...." In fact, periods spent in the sun did result in a rapid improvement in the state of my skin; pimples and blackheads dried up like sunflowers, cysts disappeared, and areas of tanned normal looking skin would appear between the scars left from Dr L's invasive activities. But these respites were short lived, and within a few days of returning to the confinement of the school rooms, the map of acne would reappear.

This period of acne, which lasted for six to seven years was not life threatening or terribly painful. But it certainly tested the resilience of my personality, with the disappointment week after week, month after month, and year after year that it was just not going away. It was also a true test of belief in the medical system. This was a condition which did not require erudite scientific articles to attest to the effectiveness of treatment in large double-blind controlled trials. Every new lump and pustule was evidence that the current treatment was ineffective.

In later years my wife would testify that she found the scars from the acne and Dr L's gouging quite attractive, but I do not think that compensated for the years of misery. So what had I learnt from these years of bad acne? Firstly, that even a non-fatal and non-painful or debilitating condition can have quite an effect on the mental status of an individual, particularly an adolescent. Secondly, I learnt that the solution for some problems (maybe most) takes a long time to come around. And in the waiting period, doctors, including specialists in the field will try many things that have not really proven their efficacy, and might even be dangerous. I was to have my thyroid gland checked regularly after the radiation delivered to my face, due to the known relationship between radiation and the development of thyroid cancer. Thirdly, even though the good treatment for acne had not been discovered during my period of suffering, as puberty ended, the skin slowly settled down on its own, with only the map of tiny scars and irregular skin folds to attest to the traumatic acne history.

Most skin pathology is not taken too seriously by medical students or medical practitioners. For most problems, the old adage, thrown around at medical school, if it's wet dry it, and if it's dry wet it, seemed to work. During medical school training, Dermatology as a specialty was never taken very seriously. Maybe this was due to the relative paucity of juicy pathology in the skin, or perhaps relating to its truly superficial place in the human body. Only following a lecture on malignant melanoma would we come alive, but even then, most of the limelight was left for the plastic surgeons who dealt with the suspicious lesions (and they were, after all, surgeons), leaving the dermatologists preoccupied with some rashes, plaques, blotches and of course the cosmetic cosmos of acne vulgaris.

I have had a long list of more serious medical problems in my life, but acne was certainly my first encounter with a chronic disorder, resistant to treatment, with significant psychosocial effects. I realise now that the understanding of the disease, at the time I was experiencing it, was still minimal and mainly descriptive, naming the different types of blemishes, furuncles and cysts seen. The role of bacteria, understanding the role of hormones and chemical compounds in eliciting the disease, was still to come. Although there was an understanding a familial predisposition to this disease exits, only today, as with almost every disease, the role of genes in the disease's development is unfolding. Two of my three children developed my type of multi-lesion acne, and within a relatively short period of time were treated with new drugs, the Retinoids. These halted the course of the disease so my children could enjoy smooth, unscarred faces and little serious suffering.

From time to time, I still reflect back on my acne period, particularly thinking about some of the young ladies who agreed to date me, and would encounter a face covered with the ravages of acne. I don't remember any screaming or running away, but I do wonder how often the polite refusal to consider another date was related to this early chronic affliction.

I certainly think my self-image was severely damaged by this period. This was a time when I perceived I was simply ugly, the ugliness being at its worst during the massive outbreaks of pustules and cysts all over my body, and persisting as I viewed the resulting scars, marking the battlefield forever. I never viewed myself as particularly handsome, but I think that up to adolescence and the acne I felt quite comfortable with what I saw in the mirror. Indeed the uncontrollable curliness of my hair annoyed me and I would have liked to be a few centimeters taller, but I saw myself as reasonable. During and following the acne period I decided that I was, well, simply ugly. The grooves and tracks adorning my face as an ongoing memory of my battle with acne had changed me for life. And then, just as it came, it was over. Suddenly, I could shave without opening bleeding pustules and I could look in the mirror each morning and see a normal face with no new red, yellow, or black bumps to welcome me. I could stop cleaning my face morning and night, could stop visiting the dermatologist, and even found myself ready to try and date girls again. Now if I failed to achieve my amorous goals, I had to find more intrinsic things to blame.

AN ACHING BACK

The return to Israel after three years of residency training in the USA was a stressful period to say the least. Firstly, there was the issue of whether this was a sane decision. Most of my colleagues who had reached the United States for further training had remained there and found excellent positions. The fact our medical training had taken place under the apartheid regime did not count against us. We were still recognized as products of an excellent medical school. Nonetheless, and with two young daughters the youngest born only six weeks before our return, my wife and I decided to take the plunge and return home to Israel. Arrangements for shipping home our American acquired possessions were carried out from my wife's hospital bed following the birth, while I negotiated my new job in Be'er Sheva. A frontier-type city, in the south of the country on the border of the desert, where I had chosen the position based on the attraction of a new medical school due to open there.

Shortly after our return, I rented a Volkswagen Beetle a marked change from the huge 1967 Dodge which we had driven in Chicago for three years. I planned to travel from my in-laws apartment near Tel Aviv, where we had set up temporary accommodation to Be'er Sheva, in order to meet my new boss and work environment. These details are relevant to my ensuing medical saga. I reached Be'er Sheva after a two hour journey and spent the day meeting my new colleagues in the hospital. During the day I noticed some twinges of pain in my lower back, which by the time I returned to Tel Aviv in the evening hours had become more intense. There was little time to worry about this new phenomenon as I joined the evening ritual of bathing the girls and preparing them for bed. We then sat down as usual for the evening meal prepared efficiently by my mother-in-law, who took the food preparation task as a serious duty.

At the end of the meal I rose from my seat and felt a stab of pain at the bottom of my back. I staggered to the sofa to rest for a few moments until the pain subsided, and then decided to proceed directly to bed. I began to lift myself from the horizontal position I was in and now experienced a new pain, the likes of which I had not only never experienced before but also I did not believe that the body could produce. The pain was shearing, vice-like, burning, and frankly terrifying. This was clearly something bad I thought, nothing benign could hurt this much. A tumour of the spinal cord? A malignant mass in the muscle? The pain of appendicitis had been bad but was a mild twinge compared to this blinding, gripping, paralysing blaze. I slept fitfully, peed in a bottle and waited for morning, letting time take its course. But time had decided that on this occasion it would provide no solace; trying to get up in the morning resulted in another primordial scream as I collapsed back on the bed. The doctor had become patient. An ambulance was called and I was transported to the hospital.

I was trundled into the emergency room, a familiar scenario from my internship at the same hospital a few years earlier. The orthopaedic resident approached me and I immediately requested that my supervisor from my orthopaedic experience in my internship be called, but I was abruptly informed that "Dr R would not leave the operating room to see an ex-intern with low back pain". I was a little miffed that my case was not receiving the expert attention necessary in severe pathology of the back. "We'd better admit him" said the orthopaedic resident to the nurse, and I was relieved to find myself bouncing on a stretcher on the way to the orthopaedic ward. No one seemed very concerned about the young doctor with *Low Back Pain*, which I attributed to the cultural lack of empathy of Israeli doctors for patients with bad diseases. I donned the blue pyjamas slowly, moving with terror of another stab of pain, and lay awaiting the decision regarding my fate. Immediate surgery? Radiotherapy and chemotherapy first? "Sorry Doc, nothing much to do here, it's far too advanced..." What a way to return home to start a career, and take the next steps of life with two young children.

But reality was far less dramatic. A bored and tired intern placed an IV in my arm and mumbled something about a trial of ACTH (a cortisone related drug) to my query regarding the procedure. Then, the nurse pushing the medicine cart between the beds placed two pills in my hand. The young doctor who turned patient asked, "Why Valium?" The answer came soon enough. By the time my wife arrived to visit me in the evening, I was smiling at all around me between periods of dozing off into a twilight zone, protecting me from the pain of muscular spasm and the traumas of re-entry into Israeli society. I was in a state closest to that of being stoned I had ever been. Realizing that I did not have some aggressive spinal disease my wife was not amused.

I was still in pain but now it was confined to the process of getting up and trying to move around. Getting to standing position became a serious life challenge - the moment that my spine reached some point of no return between lying down and sitting the stabs of fiery pain tore into my lower back, challenging even the thought of moving further. But by the following morning I could achieve the goal of reaching the bathroom, and the sweet enveloping waves of Valium on returning to bed compensated for the short period of pain during rising and walking.

This was also a moment of truth for me, to realise that not only was I not suffering from a terminal disease but also I was not even an interesting case. The ward round each morning was a short affair compared with the rounds on the paediatric wards in Chicago or Israel where the very essence of the round was the opportunity to review the notes in the chart, the laboratory and x-ray results, and show off one's knowledge of the problem to colleagues. The orthopaedic surgeons were another tribe. Marching into the ward at 7 am (at least they did not wake the patients because hospital routine demanded that the night nursing staff hand over the ward to the day staff well before that. Meaning, lights were switched on at around four thirty am), they strode from bed to bed with the senior resident mumbling a few sentences next to each bed. "Still has a fever", the attending surgeon snapping, "Change the antibiotic", or "Get an internist". As far as I remember they did not even pause next to my bed.

Later, when my head had cleared a little from the Valium, did I realise that I was in fact a VIP admission and that acute low back pain cases were usually sent home with the Valium and painkillers. Another reason I was admitted was that this particular Dr R was conducting a research protocol regarding the use of ACTH (a steroid hormone) for back pain. In those days there were no ethical committees to govern the carrying out of research on patients in wards. Agreement to participation was implicit with the reasoning that if the doctor was smart enough to research the problem, it was obvious that you agreed to be a part of it.

After three days I was home. I was much rested post intensive Valium therapy but mobility was still a major issue. Even getting upright or walking a few steps were major issues to be faced, not to mention my two infant daughters who were expecting to be lifted in my arms. I began to understand how one can learn to fear pain, the fear being as miserable as the pain itself. For the first time in my life I was experiencing a chronic disability, understanding what it is like not being able to perform the functions taken for granted each day. How long could I postpone going to the bathroom at night, to avoid having to stand upright? Could I learn to sleep with a distended bladder till morning?

Before leaving the hospital, I had a brief encounter with a physical therapist and received some cursory advice about walking with a stick and trying to lie on my side. But as I was to learn on other occasions in life, the ultimate rehabilitator of the body is oneself. The common household broom became my lifeline, always in clutching distance of my hand for the nocturnal excursion. I learnt to roll over on my side, pick up the broom, hold on to it as if my life depended on it, and press it hard downward to rise to sitting position - stage one, and then move to standing position - stage two. If there was some slight hitch in either of the stages, hell's fury would be released in my vertebral column as the inflamed disc was massaged between the two vertebrae on either side.

The other challenge related to family mobility, involving the shining new station wagon purchased in honor of the journey home to Israel. It was the state-of-the-art German technology, a glittering gold colour attesting to its individuality. But it was still a car, and therefore required two basic physiologic functions in dealing with it either as driver or passenger. One had to sit down in the car on entering, and the ultimate horror, one had to stand up in order to exit. No one had ever described this to me in lectures at medical school. We had learnt about many complex orthopaedic problems, had been questioned in our examinations about complex fractures of various bones and joint diseases, but nobody had described a simple thing like the pain of getting out of a car during a bout of acute low back pain. Only many years later did I learn about low back pain being the most common ailment affecting mankind. And now, I was learning through personal experience what it means to place your weight on your legs after sitting in a car, needing a broom to serve as the magic wand to prevent the agony of bearing weight on the lower back, and standing upright.

I began physical therapy with an experienced senior physical therapist to help the process of rehabilitation, and discovered a lesson in the fickleness of clinical medicine. "Keep your back convex", was the message given to me. I was told to lie on my side with my back rounded and to try and sit the same way. Some years later I learnt that the theory had been reversed one hundred and eighty degrees. The way to manage and prevent LBP is by maintaining the lower back in a position that could be achieved by positioning a cushion in the small of the back when sitting and most important when, driving a car.

Even today, though I have had no serious episode of low back pain for more than thirty years, I will only buy a European car having found that the seats of Japanese cars do not provide the necessary low back support. A journey in the most luxurious Japanese car invariably ends with twinges of pain in the lower back and the leg. I was given sets of exercises to strengthen the stomach muscles and was stretched on a table to release pressure on my spinal column. This low back pain attack that started as an acute episode ruled my life for at least a year, reminding me of its presence during every car journey or period of prolonged sitting at a desk.

Over the years I have encountered dozens of friends and acquaintances who have experienced the LBP syndrome, for many it became chronic with recurring attacks. There is no question that chronic pain, of which LBP is probably the most common, disturbs the quality of life to a degree few can understand. Pain is not simply a sensation sent from a nerve to the brain but a sensation that resets the way the brain perceives the world, an ultimate determinate of a feeling of wellbeing. Many of these people have fallen under the surgeon's knife, after despairing of medicine being able to relieve their suffering, and have remained with their pain after surgery. Others have slowly recovered over time with varying degrees of residual pain.

Because of its frequency, the fickleness of its course and the vivid memory of the worst pain I have ever experienced, low back pain remains a fascinating clinical entity for me. I enjoyed lecturing students at all levels showing them CT scans of patients with LBP revealing horrendous changes in the structure of the discs between the vertebrae with no pain, and on the other hand there are patients with intractable back pain whose CT's show little or no change at all. The lesson to be learnt is that a good clinician will never rely on the clinical picture, a CT or laboratory results alone, to reach a diagnosis.

Time and again we learn that even with all the technologic advances in medicine, the diagnosis will depend on a thorough clinical history together with the clinical examination, and the imaging and laboratory data. The special nature of the LBP entity is further complicated, or simplified depending how one looks at it, by the fact that LBP increases during periods of mental stress. Could my attack of acute LBP have been related to my life events at that time? Perhaps returning to Israel after three years in the USA with two young children, moving to a new place, and taking up a new professional posting constituted enough stress to burst out as an attack of LBP? This was certainly one of the first major tests for me as a patient that also helped me, in the years to come, to reflect on how I deal with my body in these situations. Certainly, my level of empathy for anyone who complains about low back pain has been high since then. I could never have felt the same way just through reading books or hearing lectures. I felt good when I could look people in the eye, as they tried to impress upon me the degree of their suffering and say, "Hey, I've been there".

The issue of low back pain is a typical touch point in medicine today between technology and emotions. It really depends on where one is focusing, on the back or the pain? The tendency of modern medicine is to focus on a specific organ, in a specific area, and decide whether the intervention will be medical, usually involving medications, or surgical - suggesting that a surgeon's knife can either remove a pathology or construct an anatomical solution to the problem. Other therapists who are frequently involved include physical therapists or chiropractors who have a specific philosophy and interventions regarding management of spinal pathology. One approach is that sufferers from pain in the lower back will embark on a journey of progressive levels of painkillers and muscle relaxants, undergo series of treatments from physical therapists, and then after various periods of suffering will decide that only surgery will rescue them from their misery. All attention is directed to correcting the area of the back that is causing pain.

A second approach is to focus on pain perception as the primary problem and look at low back pain as a predominant pain issue.

Any kind of pain is unpleasant and has its own special aspects. Low back pain is a pain connected with one of the human being's most basic needs - the need to move around, to walk, get up, sit down, lie down, or drive a car. When most of these activities are accompanied by pain life becomes one big pain so to speak, and it is easy to understand why chronic back pain leads to depression.

My experience with a severe attack of LBP as a young man has maintained my interest in the problem as a physician (even though low back pain does not feature as a paediatric problem). It serves as a beautiful model for the fickleness of medical doctrine. Bed rest and slow mobilization as the cornerstones of care have been replaced by a policy of minimal rest and keeping moving. A mainstay of traditional medicine was challenged when medical science found that here was a condition that the prognosis for most people was improved if they did not don pyjamas and climb into bed. But instead force themselves to limp around, do some exercises to strengthen their muscles of the abdomen, and take some simple pain killers.

Some rest is necessary, but the body that keeps moving stays healthy. This policy has affected not only back pain sufferers but has become part of cardiac rehabilitation and post-surgery routine as well, and both the work force and patients have benefited from this approach that challenged tradition.

There is still an amazing lack of knowledge regarding probably the most common affliction of mankind. We know a lot of things that can trigger back pain, but for most people it is a bolt from the blue with a high likelihood of recurrence. Also, there is a lot of quackery relating to the condition, with the amount of potential healers increasing as the numbers of sufferers continue to grow. Nevertheless, a treatment approach requiring the active participation of the sufferer is a refreshing message for medicine today. Reminding sufferers that potential healers whether family practitioners, orthopaedic surgeons, acupuncturists or shamans can err, as they are all only human and at the end you the sufferer have your destiny in your own hands.

JAUNDICED

My internship year was a rotating style internship at Sheba hospital, a large teaching hospital in the Tel Aviv area. Also, in addition to the time spent in different wards in order to gain wide experience (internal medicine, surgery, paediatrics, and other clinical specialties), I was required to spend a two month period in Israel's periphery. This was part of Sheba hospital's national commitment to help the small peripheral hospitals, which always suffered from a dearth of trained personnel, both junior and senior. I was sent to the hospital in Safed, a small town, situated above the Sea of Galilee. I was the intern in the internal medicine ward, with plenty of time off to spend travelling around and touring the pretty landscape. The department head, an experienced physician, made sure that the routine workload was finished by twelve am allowing for a leisurely lunch in the hospital canteen, and a good afternoon break (the traditional Shlafstunde[3]), before returning for another quick round in the late afternoon.

I was thoroughly enjoying this relaxed routine, a welcome break from the demanding routine at Sheba hospital, when I suddenly felt distinctly off-colour. The main expression of this "feeling ill" was a feeling of nausea causing me to recoil from any food, or even the smell of something cooking. The problem was that the smells of lunch cooking in the hospital kitchen traveled through the hospital corridors and wards just as we would begin the morning rounds, causing me to focus on my nausea instead of on the diagnostic dilemmas of the patients. I also lost my taste for cigarettes which should have given me a clue regarding my problem. Doctors smoked freely at this time, and I was strongly addicted, needing my first cigarette immediately with my morning coffee. After two or three days of feeling ill, I was told by one of my colleagues on the round that I was looking "a little yellow". I was instructed to lie down, blood and urine specimens were taken from me, and I was informed that I had jaundice, or more correctly *Infectious*

---

3. Afternoon resting time (Siesta). Literary German - an hour's sleep.

Hepatitis, and was ordered to be hospitalized in the ward.

Within a few hours I had changed my tailored white safari coat and stethoscope for the dusky blue pyjamas with the words Ministry of Health emblazoned on the back, given to all patients, and was lying in a bed in one of the rooms. Hepatitis was a very common condition in Israel in those days, a condition not yet fully understood, except for its high infectivity, particularly in crowded institutions such as the military. Also, there was not much to do about it, except monitor the level of jaundice and wait for it to pass. So there I was, rapidly moving from the role of doctor to one of a patient, which was confusing both to me and to some of the patients on the ward. I remember clearly coming to the dining area on the first evening of hospitalisation, and sitting down next to an elderly gentleman from the ward who had been under my care. I had taken a blood specimen from him that same morning. By his expression I could tell he was clearly puzzled to see me sit next to him, another blue clad resident of the ward. I tried to explain with a smile that "Yes, I am the same doctor who had attended to him earlier in the day", but I think it was too overwhelming for him, as he turned away and continued to slurp his soup with a slight shake of the head.

This episode of jaundice was short. The values of bilirubin[4] which reflected the severity of the

---

4. The yellow breakdown and clearance of the body's aged red blood cells containing hemoglobin

disease rapidly dropped back to normal. Within two or three days I felt and looked fully recovered and was discharged. The next day I was back on the ward in my intern role, my patient from dinner a few days back still hospitalized. As the morning round reached his bed he fixed me with a bewildered gaze, probably questioning his own memory as the cause for his confusion. Doctor turning patient and then doctor again was probably a more difficult explanation to reason with than just questioning the fallibility of his brain. I have often reflected on this first experience of moving from being the doctor to becoming the patient.

What is most vivid in my memory even after forty years is how I wished that I would be treated as a patient and not as a medical colleague. The moment that my jaundice was diagnosed and I was told to check in as a patient, I was pretty much left to make my own decisions. The medical staff would pass by my bed with a smile, muttering something about my bilirubin level, and move on to the next bed. I needed some explanation and reassurance regarding the diagnosis, I needed a Dr C to say to me "Stay in bed three more days and do not eat foods a. b and c". Instead, I was the doctor. The modern day "Physician heal thyself[5]". This episode passed quickly. So quickly that it was a questionable case of hepatitis, probably not eligible for more than a definition of being "a little liverish". But the next episode left little doubt.

---

5. Luke 4:23

My wife and I with our two young daughters were off to visit my parents in South Africa. Much excitement, planning, and getting organized with two little girls aged four and two years. The day before we left Israel I was called in to see the neighbour's son who was sick, and very yellow. A few questions revealed the lack of appetite, the lethargy, and the dark urine. He was yellow as yellow could be, and I quickly confirmed the diagnosis of jaundice. Did I wash my hands properly after palpating his abdomen? And then we were off to be swept away in the family embrace and memories of childhood. The floods of memories and nostalgia began with the journey home from the airport; the return to the house I grew up and lived in until graduating from medical school and leaving for Israel, T-bone steaks and papayas, peanut butter and peppermint crisp chocolate bars, and continued with the warm welcome from the house staff who had played such an important role in my life.

Then came the day when the first one and then the second child came down with a fever and vomiting. Things only began to connect a few days later when my wife complained of lethargy and nausea, then the dark yellow-brown urine confirming the probable line of infection from the neighbour via the children to her. Hepatitis was indeed a highly infectious disease. Still, I was not expecting to be the ultimate target of the virus path. Again I suddenly lost my taste for cigarettes and then for the foods of my youth. The delicious fish, lamb chops and biltong[6] became foreign to me, my voracious appetite for the tastes of my childhood vanished. Instead of drooling saliva at the sight of Johanna's (our cook) wondrous roast chicken with crispy roast potatoes waves of nausea seized me. I was next in the chain of infectious hepatitis, the virus that attacked the liver causing the main visible sign of the disease - jaundice. I was optimistic.

The children recovered from their mild illness barely showing jaundice, the usual story with small children, and my wife despite a few days of suffering from pruritis - a severe itching associated with jaundice, soon lost her yellow hew and within a week was looking her former healthy self. So I was not overly concerned when I saw my yellow urine becoming progressively darker. A few days of the vacation had been spoiled, but hopefully there would be a few remaining days to enjoy the fleshpots of my youth before returning to Israel.

By the time I was put to bed, my wife and daughters were on the mend returning to normal function. The decision was made - they would return on the scheduled flight and I would postpone my flight for a few days. I lay back in my bed following their departure, feeling the subtle role change from husband and father back to being the baby of my parents, the title always attached by my mother to the younger of her two sons. I was back to taking

---

6. South African dried cured meat, similar to the American beef jerky.

orders, and regressed to being the sick son, Dr C's patient. The paediatrician who had recently returned from Chicago, the Young Turk helping set up a new medical school in the desert of Israel was a distant memory. It seemed quite fortunate, at least for me, that I did not have to feel guilty about not helping with the children or with washing the dishes. Fickle fate had placed those issues now six thousand miles away, so I might as well lie back and enjoy the trip in the time machine to a Johannesburg childhood.

The positive scenario that had been embraced began to fade. As each day passed, the feeling of nausea did not subside and the colour of my skin moved progressively from pale yellow through darker shades reaching a true orange hue, the whites of my eyes now a stark yellow. The urine was dark sepia, my stools pale grey. This was a technicolour disease. As the illness progressed, and it was clear that it was not going to end in a few days, Dr C was called in to take over from the patient-doctor. I was happy to release myself from being my own doctor, trying to understand, and to explain to my worried parents why the mild disease experienced by my family was behaving so strangely within my body. Dr C had no trouble relating to me as he always had.

The journey in my time capsule to my youth had Dr C ascending the stairs and walking into my room, looking confident and professional in an immaculate jacket, perfectly pressed slacks, silk tie, carrying the ultimate symbol of the doctor in this environment - the doctor's bag. This was no throw bag like the one I used, stashed with a stethoscope and reflex hammer, but rather a large Cadillac, which opened into two compartments, each stuffed with instruments, medicines, syringes and prescription pads. The interaction with me was strictly doctor-patient oriented, with a few moments at the end allowed for professional banter regarding the diagnostic thinking and treatment plan. This was purely for information, while it was absolutely clear that Dr C was in charge, irrespective of my status in the profession.

I think this was the real strength of the general practitioner in South Africa of those days. He was the unquestioned manager of the patient, not only in the eyes of the patient, but also in the eyes of any specialist that might be involved in the patient's care. The fact that nothing was done to the patient without the knowledge and assent of the GP gave him a special aura and authority, a true status of the responsible healer. A famous neurosurgeon might perform a major operation on a patient, a prominent cardiologist might diagnose the nature of a heart problem, but the ultimate coordinator of healing and the responsibility for the patient's health rested with Dr C. Thus it was no surprise that I was ready to shed the role of physician and sink into the role of the patient, and no less a surprise that Dr C had no problem managing the doctor in bed. There was no other way to do things. Dr C called the private laboratory to arrange the tests, called the pharmacy to order medicines, instructed my mother regarding dietary precautions and then snapped shut the medical bag and swiftly moved out of the room on his way to the next visit. I was safe, everything was under control.

My appetite returned, a sure sign that I must be on the mend. But this did not seem to be holding true, as I began to shed kilograms of weight and my skin developed increasing shades of deep orange. Huge amounts of calories were being taken in, as I witnessed my body slimming daily. The laboratory tests showed the classic picture of infectious hepatitis, high levels of liver enzymes indicating liver damage together with an ongoing rise in the level of bilirubin, the pigment responsible for the yellowing of the skin. There was no treatment, just the necessity to monitor the damage to the liver until things would begin to turn around. But my episode of infectious jaundice, this most common disease, was not behaving in the usual manner. The jaundice was not receding, the enzymes levels stayed sky high, the weight loss progressed, and there was more to come.

I now became aware of a strange sensation under my skin, a sensitivity to touch which then progressed to a slight itch. "Yes", explained Dr C reminding me that my wife had also experienced this common symptom of jaundice known as pruritis, literally - an itching. I had not paid much attention to my wife when she described her itch, and smiled condescendingly as she would lie on the shag carpet and roll around to soothe it. Womanly hysteria was probably at the back of my mind. But now, as I experienced this progressive pruritis I begged forgiveness from the Gods for my lack of empathy. The pruritis became an invader, an enemy that I faced with terror and fear. I could not tolerate clothes on my skin, the warm bath which I thought would soothe, only aggravated the itch. I rolled on the carpet at all hours of night and day, wore only short cotton undershorts belonging to my father, a skinny, orange apparition with yellow eyes contrasted against baggy white shorts, a pseudo-Mahatma Gandhi looking back at me in the mirror. I had lost many kilograms in weight, and was surprised that when I sat in the bathtub I was able to feel my pubic bones, no longer covered with a healthy cushion of fat.

The bilirubin reached levels which caused even the poker-faced professional Dr C to respond with a momentary look of bewilderment, mixed with concern. This case of hepatitis now filed outside of his range of experience with the disease. He suggested that the time had come for a consultation, and suggested Dr K, a liver specialist who had been one of my teachers in medical school, a brilliant young academic who even then was clearly marked for the top. He did not usually see private consultations as he was a senior consultant at NEH (Non-European Hospital, the euphemistic abbreviation for the hospital for the black population, adjacent to The Gen, the general whites-only hospital). He readily agreed to see me, as a professional colleague, and said he would stop by on Sunday afternoon, not a usual time for a consultation.

He duly arrived attired in white shorts and shirt on the way to his squash game. I will never forget my sudden feeling of despair as I stared at his pink hands and white clothes as he examined my yellow stained body, feeling like a foreign entity in this world of the white. He was brisk and professional, demonstrating the interaction characteristic of physicians who had spent their days working with the "other" population, a population with no medical services except for emergency rooms and hospitals catering for non-whites, those who had little right to anything under the apartheid regime. Doctors working in this system frequently did not establish the communication skills so required and used by doctors working in the private practices of the white opulent suburbs, but rather developed a more veterinary approach to their medicine. He thrust his hand into my abdomen, pummeled my liver and spleen, and proceeded to say a few sentences to me, explaining that this was still a "typical though severe" picture of infectious hepatitis, and he did not see a need for further tests.

And as it often happens, a few days after the consultant had been called in, I started to feel better, my mood improved, and the bilirubin levels began to fall. I began to gain weight and boarded the plane back to Tel Aviv some weeks later, still thin and very orange, but on the mend. My Israeli colleagues did not react with great surprise to my story, the disease being very prevalent in Israel including the more severe cases. Eventually, an internist colleague did help in solving the mystery of my case. He suggested I had a genetic disorder known as Gilbert's syndrome, characterized by a problem with bilirubin disposal. This could explain the mild case of jaundice experienced in earlier years, and the extremely high level of jaundice in the current episode. I immediately felt better. The knowledge concerning why something had happened helped to instill a feeling of some control over the situation. But the saga of Gilbert's syndrome and my liver was still to be continued.

Some seven years later, I transferred my young family with me to Boston for a sabbatical fellowship in child development. I blossomed during that year as I acquired new professional knowledge and skills, accompanied by social and cultural experiences which contributed so much to a sabbatical. I could spend time with patients, there were no norms to meet, and I was exposed to an amazing number of extremely smart people, including some idols whose names I knew only from books and journals. The sabbatical atmosphere was enriching and rewarding, and as the end of the year approached I realised how great an effect this experience had imprinted on me. While busy in last minute purchases and packing before the return journey home, I began to feel some stomach pain. It took a little time to dawn on me that I was in fact experiencing a type of recurrent pain which was quite severe. I swallowed antacids[7] and the pain

7. A substance used for neutralizing stomach acidity and relieving heartburn.

would subside each time within a few hours so I did not give it much thought. After three or four (or five, or six, or twenty?) of these episodes I decided that maybe the time has come to see a specialist.

The gastroenterologist received me in the polite and professional way I would expect of a specialist, without giving any special attention to the fact I was a physician. After taking a history and feeling my abdomen, he sat me down at his desk and said, "You know this could be gallbladder disease?" I had not even thought of this during my self-assessment of my problem. I thought back to our lectures on gallbladder disease at medical school, the mnemonic of the "Fat, Female at Fifty" who typically suffered from gallstone disease. I certainly did not fit in there, but I respected the expert opinion and promised to follow this up when I got back home to Israel in a few months' time, a promise I failed to keep. I never did initiate anything further. I returned to the treadmill of professional and daily life without the friendly parachute of the sabbatical. There was no time for bodily cares while children were being settled back in schools and my wife and I were adjusting to the new work pressures.

And then came the reminder that said that I really had to DO something. We were returning from a visit to friends on a kibbutz one Saturday evening. As I drove along the road between Beit Shemesh and Be'er Sheva the familiar pain began in my stomach. I ignored it as much as I could, but at a certain point it was clear that there was no going on. I stopped the car at the side of the road and lay down outside writhing in a spasm of agonizing, debilitating pain while my wife and children watched with puzzlement and concern from the car windows. And then, after ten minutes it was gone. I stood up and sat back in the passenger seat as my wife continued the drive homeward. I stared ahead pondering the experience until the penny dropped. I laughed at myself for not realizing the obvious before - I had just experienced a classic attack of gallbladder colic. A stone was obstructing the tube from the gallbladder to the gut, setting in motion an involuntary muscular process in the wall of the tube, causing the awful pain which disappeared only when the obstruction had passed.

I knew the theory from Professor Du Plessis's surgery lectures from fifteen years earlier, "Picture trying to squeeze a golf ball through a straw". For me it was clear that those suffering from gallstones need not imagine it, they experience it firsthand. Although I was not fat, fifty or female, it seemed I had gallbladder stones. Now, I needed confirmation.

The next day I presented myself to the ultrasound department at my hospital. With the picture clearly documenting a collection of small stones in my gallbladder, I returned for a brief consultation with one of the surgeons. "So, what next?" I asked the surgeon. "We take it out". Surgeons really don't talk a lot, and when they clearly see that the knife is the solution words are even more superfluous in their eyes. It was a strange sensation. Here I was feeling perfectly healthy, and being told that I had to schedule major surgery for myself. It is different if in hospital, sick and clearly a patient when the surgeon says he must operate. Next, I was walking back to my child development clinic to see patients, to attend meetings, and then return home to help feed the children and hear about everybody's day. And I had to fix a date for having an organ taken out of my body.

On the day before surgery, I spent the morning pretending to work in my clinic and tried to keep myself busy until four pm when I duly presented myself in the surgery ward for admission. I was now a pre-op patient. I had a light meal and from then it was NPO (nothing by mouth). The next morning, while expecting to be early on the list, I discovered that my doctor's status had not helped me, as there were emergencies filling the operating rooms. I spent until two pm staring at the ceiling and pretending to be calm. Finally, I was placed on a stretcher and bounced to the floor of the operating rooms, where there was a further wait in a small side room full of nursing equipment. I remember an overwhelming feeling of loneliness and impending doom as I lay in that room, wondering if I would awake from the anaesthetic to see my family again. By the time I was wheeled into the operating room I was in a state of extreme anxiety, wondering why this healthy person was doing this to himself. I was greeted by a colleague, a senior anaesthetist, who quietly tried to reassure me as he deftly inserted an intravenous line in my arm, and then those confusing few moments before total blackness again.

Recovery from this surgical foray was uneventful. My cheerful surgeon said the gallbladder was full of "mud", the meaning of which was not quite clear at the time. When it came to changing the bandage covering my wound I was surprised to see a ten centimeter long scar lying under my ribcage. The cheerful surgeon then explained that there were many adhesions inside my abdomen, probably dating back to my earlier appendix surgery, which required a large cut to enable him to view the area. I still have a slight suspicion that some medical students were observing my surgery, and when they complained they were having difficulty viewing, the surgeon simply increased the length of the cut. One thing is certain – I had just missed out on a major surgical technologic advance. Shortly after undergoing this operation endoscopic surgery began taking center stage. Since, gallbladder surgery, like most surgery in the abdomen, is performed through two or more small holes which allow for an endoscope to be inserted and the offending organ removed without the need for long anaesthetics and huge cuts. This is again proof that any dogma will change with time. Our revered professor of surgery at medical school would launch into tirades regarding the dangers of keyhole surgery, referring to the fashionable surgeons who would remove an appendix through a small cut to ensure that their patient would be able to continue wearing a bikini with unblemished skin over the tummy.

I was still not sure why I had succumbed to gallstone disease. The description of the stones as "mud" also contrasted with the classic gallstones which were much larger. One day, the internist who was familiar with my history of prolonged jaundice casually mentioned that in patients with Gilbert's disease, in addition to a tendency to jaundice, there could be a hemolytic process (breakdown of red blood cells), resulting in the formation of small stones in the gallbladder. I liked the fact that I could now connect my bad experience with jaundice and my recent stomach pains to a minor genetic problem, regarding disposal of bile pigments, which later caused gallbladder disease that was surgically treatable.

I had reached the age of forty. I had experienced and survived two episodes of abdominal surgery and had two most impressive scars over my abdomen, always a topic for conversation at the sea or poolside. My liver has continued to remind me of its existence over the years. Taking a few doses of the common over-the-counter drug paracetamol (Tylenol) will send my liver enzyme levels soaring, and induce anxiety in any physician seeing those results. At the time of my gallbladder surgery, I had requested that the surgeon take a small piece of the liver to send for biopsy. The pathology report of that specimen was normal. So I knew I did not suffer from a serious chronic disease of this critical organ, but it was still sending me signals later in life that at more advanced molecular levels all was not completely well. I was also learning from my own body, that just as there may be a sensitivity of an organ to disease or dysfunction, there also seems to be much resilience to damage in our complicated networks of body organs.

The recovery from a severe infection and blockage of bile flow, the continued normal life after removing the gallbladder, or the rapid return of liver function to normal after stopping a drug, all helped me strengthen my confidence in the ability of our bodies to fight back. The trouble was that mostly this fight did not seem to be under our control but rather determined by a primal genetic programming of all bodily functions, which included the tendency to develop malfunction happily together with an ability for self-righting.

My path through liver and gallbladder disease had taught me a lot about experiencing symptoms. It was one thing to study symptoms of liver disease or gallbladder colic in a textbook and practice the learning while taking histories from patients. Personal experience was a different story all together. The nausea and loss of appetite from liver disease, the indescribable crescendo-decrescendo pain of gallbladder colic, and the despair from itching that did not respond to simple scratching, the pruritis of bile duct obstruction, opened up my world of trying to better understand patients' symptoms. No five minute routine list of questions regarding symptomatology would ever truly convey what a patient with these kinds of symptoms is experiencing. How much more difficult is trying to understand feelings of depression or anxiety, or the young child's experience of high fever?

I have had the privilege of entering the profession of medicine in the era when doctors finally had proof that certain tools and technologies work. From simple medicines to reduce pain and fever, antibiotics which cured infectious diseases, and then the discovery of medicines that could really treat cancer as well as techniques that allowed new organs to be transplanted when old ones had failed. Prior to this era, the doctor could not do much more than listen and comfort with no real science in his hands. My experiences had allowed me to continue a normal life thanks to new knowledge and exciting technologies. Luck also seemed to have been on my side, and in the years to come would be a constant player in my life.

EASTER ON HAMPSTEAD HEATH

We were nearing the end of a sabbatical year in London, another year of new experiences professionally and socially. Absorbing the wonders of the sprawling, dynamic city of London, it was a glorious spring Saturday of a long Easter weekend, and I had decided to take my thirteen-year-old son to Hampstead Heath to see the last typical English fair before we return home to Israel.

We strode from our apartment to the circle next to the entrance to the heath, well known for the landmark Jack Straw's pub, and started to cross at the pedestrian crossing. As with most such crossings in England the crossing was marked by a flashing beacon, in addition to the stripes on the road. I was lost in conversation with my son in the middle of the crossing, as I became aware of the front of a car impending on my field of vision and heard my son say something like, "Look out dad". This was followed by a sharp bump to my right knee, and then I felt myself sailing through the air before landing on the road, with my head taking an additional sharp knock. I lay for a few seconds on the ground checking that I was conscious, and performing a short review of my body parts.

In the middle of this process, I heard a high-pitched female voice chattering next to my aching head, asking my poor son "Is he alright?" Mainly to reassure my son I reached out for help in getting onto my feet, as a policeman approached and asked if he should call for an ambulance. In light of the lack of blood on the ground and the fact that I could stand, I immediately protested and said that everything was fine. But as my brain began to register the pain from the right knee I realised that maybe everything was not completely in order, and that I should be evaluated in a hospital. The owner of the high-pitched voice immediately offered to drive me to the hospital, an offer I foolishly accepted. I sat in her car with my son and then realised that her condition was less stable than mine. Starting the car she flooded the engine, and it took some calming down and advice from my son before she regained her ability to drive. On the way to the hospital she talked incessantly, aggravating my steadily worsening headache. I was relieved no further mishap had happened en route, and happily exited the car as we reached the entrance to the emergency room of the Royal Free Hospital.

I entered the ER holding on to my concerned son's arm, and stood in line to register. Easter Saturday was obviously a busy day, with patients and staff mingling and moving in the typical pattern of organized chaos in most hospital emergency rooms. At this point, in addition to the pain in my head and my knee, I began to feel slightly dizzy and decided to behave with a little more authority. So against all the rules of English decorum, particularly regarding the "sanctity of the queue", I leaned over to the clerk and said: "I'm a doctor who has been involved in a car accident", and was directed to sit among a large group of people waiting to be seen. A minute later a nurse appeared, who asked me a few questions about the event, checked my pulse and blood pressure, and shone a light in my eyes. Noting the scrapes on my forehead and legs, and that I was not feeling too well, she directed me into a wheelchair and proceeded to push me into the bowels of the emergency room. She pulled a curtain back from one of the many cubicles surrounding the central area, and pushed me inside, instructing me to move from the wheelchair to a chair in the cubicle. "I'm sorry, there are no beds, so you'll have to wait in the chair", she remarked before darting off.

At this point I was starting to feel very sore, very weak, and very dizzy, these feelings worsening by the minute as I sat uncomfortably in the upright position. Finally, the curtain was pushed aside and an extremely tired and stressed looking physician entered the cubicle. She examined me briefly after hearing the story, and sent me for an x-ray of the knee, where once more a line of patients waited patiently for the understaffed technicians.

After waiting for the x-ray to be done, and a further wait for the radiologist's report, I met the harassed doctor once more, who seemed to be the only physician on duty on this busy holiday. She reviewed the x-ray report informing me that there was no obvious injury, and I should rest a few days at home and then be re-checked by my doctor. At some point my wife arrived and took control over the situation and after three or four hours in the emergency room we made it home.

As we got back home, I suddenly remembered that we were booked to travel to Switzerland the following day for a week of skiing. I lay on my bed with the room spinning around me and my leg throbbing. Hitting the slopes in Pontresina twenty four hours later was clearly not an option. Cancellation of the trip would not only be a big disappointment for my son and older daughter who was visiting, but also a fairly big financial loss. Just as I was getting ready to break the news to my children, my wife threw out a practical solution to the problem. "You anyway have to lie and rest so you might as well do it in a nice hotel in Switzerland, and not spoil the holiday". This seemed a rational suggestion to which I readily agreed. And so the family continued packing while I lay in bed.

The next morning, after not a particularly restful night, we set off on our journey. I looked a little the worse for wear, feeling tired, weak, and dizzy with grazes over the forehead and some swelling around the eyes. The journey included a relatively short flight to Zurich from Gatwick airport, where we boarded a train to Pontresina. Despite the Swiss punctuality, this journey was long. We then moved on to progressively smaller trains, on narrower rails, as we advanced upwards in the mountains where we were joined by herds of joyful skiers. While the trains left each station on the exact second scheduled, as the seconds hand of the clocks at the stations struck 12:00, I was not aware of the need for validating the tickets before boarding each new train. Every conductor shook his head in despair at this lack of attention to Swiss precision, my bruised face and crutches having no effect on their tolerance for the ill-bred tourists.

When I disembarked at our destination with crutches, some puzzled skiers looked at me wondering how I was in this shape before even having reached the slopes. I was tired, dizzy and sore, and just wished to get to bed. On getting up in the night to reach the bathroom, I experienced significant lightheadedness which together with the painful knee made the simplest of basic tasks difficult to perform. I began to think that perhaps my body had taken a more severe beating then first perceived. But now I was here among the snowcapped peaks, so I had better make the best of it.

As daylight streamed through the windows, and

I prepared to get up and start the day, I noticed a new problem. My right knee had swelled to double the size of its partner on the left and was now very, very painful. I staggered and hopped to the nurse in the clinic after breakfast. She took one look at the knee and indicated that I must see the doctor in the village. A short taxi ride brought me to the doctor's clinic, set in a well-furnished chocolate box-like Swiss cottage. The doctor took a quick look at me and my crutches and asked me to undress. After a few jabs at the swollen, painful knee he reassured me that there was no fracture. He then proceeded to apply globs of ointment over the affected knee, followed by wrapping bandages over a splint, and instructing me to report back in two days. I realised that this was the meat and potatoes pathology for any doctor located adjacent to a popular ski area in Switzerland.

I returned to the resort ready to begin my recuperation. The family had taken off to the slopes with the appropriate teachers, and I settled myself into a comfortable chair on the verandah of the hotel with a good book in hand. This was to be my routine for the following days, only to be interrupted by meals with the family as they returned flushed and excited by their newly acquired skills on the slopes. From time to time I would be joined on the verandah by one of the skiers, limping with crutches and plaster casts, who would cheerfully tell of their falls on the slopes as they negotiated the turns on a challenging trail. I would wait for the inevitable question regarding my injury, and would sheepishly relay my history of the car accident at the pedestrian crossing on Hampstead Heath. After seeing how wimpish this story sounded up here on the glorious Swiss ski slopes, I considered making up a good yarn appropriate to the place. But decided there was too much of a chance of being revealed as a charlatan which would be even more embarrassing than the true story.

Over the following days, it became clear to me that the accident had not resulted only in a blow to the knee. As I would attempt to rise from the bed in the room the walls would begin to rotate, and I felt as if I was walking on a slow moving roller coaster, reaching out for support before an imminent fall. As I lay in bed this feeling would persist, convincing me that the knock to my head had shaken up the brain inside. I remembered that as I opened my eyes after being knocked over, I had immediately reassured myself that I was not suffering from concussion which according to my medical school training had to involve a period of loss of consciousness. But even if I did not fit the definition, clearly something had happened to the brain causing feelings of unsteadiness and dizziness.

Some years later, I was reminded about the effects of trauma more vividly following a much more serious accident. Both incidents let me reflect on lectures in surgery by our God-like professor of surgery, who talked about the effects of trauma on the body irrespective of the specific visible injuries. Later, in my internship and residency days, I learnt that the obvious injury is not always the most important one. Every patient being examined after any trauma should have a full assessment, including a careful history and examination before deciding on further tests and or treatment, procedures I had obviously missed out on during the hours spent at the London emergency room.

From my personal file of cases that taught me lessons for life, I remember being on call in the surgery unit during my internship in Israel. A child of seven years old was admitted from a car accident and because of a finding of bloody urine was referred to the urologist, who examined him in the operating room, finding a tear of the urethra - the tube allowing urine to pass from the bladder through the penis. The tear was repaired and the child was returned to the surgical ward where he remained unconscious and breathing poorly. As no intensive care unit existed in hospitals in Israel at the time, he was nursed in the surgery ward where it was decided he needed continued help with breathing, via a bag connected to the tube in his breathing pipe. I, as the intern on call, was the obvious choice to continue squeezing the bag over many hours as the child's condition slowly deteriorated until he finally died in the early morning hours.

I went home in a somber mood to try and connect with the happy atmosphere of the Independence Day celebrations. The next morning I was informed by my department head that an autopsy had been performed to ascertain the cause of death - a massive bleed into the lung. He added that had a bronchoscope been inserted into the tube leading to the lung at an early stage the child might have been saved. The bleed from the urethra had clearly been of secondary importance, though the more obvious finding immediately after the accident. A sleepless night had been spent in a futile exercise to try and save a child whose primary injury had been tragically missed.

At the ski clinic my bandages were changed every few days, the knee remaining swollen and painful, but by the time we were due to fly back to London at least the bruises and scrapes on my face had receded and I was looking pretty normal. Now was the time to get expert advice.

I was referred to a leading Harley street orthopaedic surgeon, who was in professional jargon a top "knee man". I arrived for my appointment excited at this opportunity to meet Harley street medicine first-hand, the place with a reputation for housing the best of British doctors in every specialty that existed. I entered the office and was greeted by the nurse who invited me to wait in the lavishly furnished waiting room, looking more like a Victorian parlor than a doctor's waiting room. After a few minutes of perusing the paintings on the wall and the carpets on the floor, I was ushered into Mr B's presence (British surgeons still demand to be called Mr and not Dr as a stamp of superiority, a tradition dating back to the era when a surgeon was equated with a barber, which was for some strange reason now seen as highly prestigious). Mr B welcomed me, glanced at my medical notes, and directed me to remove my pants and lie on the examination table. He pressed and squeezed my knee, measured it with a tape and swiftly commented, "Doesn't look too bad", and invited me back for follow up after some physical therapy.

I dutifully returned for two or three return examinations, which were much of the same albeit shorter than the first. I asked if there was a need for any further action regarding the knee. "Well, we might see some specific injury like a foreign body if we look inside", was his reply, indicating the possible need for arthroscopy - taking a look inside the knee joint through an endoscopic tool. "How soon could that be done?" I asked, as at this point I was involved with legal issues regarding the accident as well as approaching the date for us to return to Israel. "We could probably do you in November", he replied laconically. I paused, and then proceeded, "And if we do it privately?" "Next Monday", he flashed back with no change of expression. Here I was testing the British National Health Service, the model to all countries for accessible, affordable medicine for all. Here was the reality that when it was affordable it was accessible, the only question being "when?"

From there things moved quickly and the following Monday I presented myself to the small private hospital where I was admitted to a private, luxuriously furnished room in preparation for the procedure that evening. I remember once more the bright lights and silent efficiency of the operating room, the reassuring words of the anaesthetist as he injected me with something that had put me into a short, restful, and painless sleep. The next thing I remembered was seeing Mr B's almost smiling face saying a cheerful "Hello Basil", following which I could order a meal and then had a restful night's sleep. Woken by Mr B the following morning at 6 am, he informed me that the knee looked "Pretty good", and that he had removed a small foreign body and scraped some damaged part of the knee. And then he was gone. Off to start his day of surgery, hopefully with more interesting pathology than that of the Israeli doctor he had just visited.

I had been assured that recovery from this procedure would be rapid and painless. The only problem was that at this point I was staying with friends, as my family had returned to Israel to enable my son start the new school year. These friends had a typical Victorian house in Bayswater with my guest room on the third floor, some sixty steps up. This was mildly challenging at the best of times, but returning with the heavily bandaged and painful knee made recovery more challenging. Somehow, I managed to cope with this problem and one week later I was on a plane back home to Israel, still very conscious of a painful and rather poorly functioning knee.

Back home, I continued to limp around, returning to work and domestic life. I attached myself to a senior physical therapist who confidently assured me that various exercise and taping of the knee would ensure recovery. Sure enough, function gradually returned and my injured knee became a distant memory. Like so many other ailments, I was never quite sure what exactly happened in my knee. There was no question that a very heavy object, a motor car, had struck my knee. I know there are numerous ligaments around the knee that keep it functioning in normal and stressful situations, and there had been damage though not a total tear of those ligaments. Inside the knee there was probably some bruising, maybe a little dislodging of a fragment of the cartilage, and probably enough damage to guarantee poor functioning of the knee in my later years.

Would have things been done differently today? The orthopaedic surgeon would probably order an MRI to get a good picture of the tissues in and around the knee before the surgical procedure. This might have persuaded the surgeon that no intervention was necessary, or he might have decided to do the procedure anyway, thus covering all possibilities. So why the MRI? This is an example of the kind of issues facing the medical profession in almost every field today. How much do I need to investigate to be sure? Can I ever be completely sure? And probably the doctor of today is also thinking: *does this MRI or arthroscopy justify the expense to the system*?

Apart from the medical lessons from this episode with my knee, the accident also exposed me to medicolegal issues which accompanied the accident. The facts were quite simple in my eyes. I had been knocked over by a moving car, walking on a pedestrian crossing clearly marked on the street, and the flashing beacon alongside. There was also a policeman, on the beat standing nearby the crossing, who had witnessed the event and suggested calling an ambulance. By refusing the offer of an ambulance I probably harmed my chances of recognition as a severe accident victim. Arriving in the company of ambulance attendants at the emergency room, instead of hobbling in alongside my son, would have been a far more impressive entry as a trauma patient. This was brought home to me when I received a letter from the Hampstead police some weeks after the accident, informing me that they did not find any reason to pursue the circumstances of my accident. I saw this as a blatant failure of justice but was persuaded by my lawyer not to pursue the issue, assuring me that I would not achieve much.

The other experience with the justice system in England occurred one day when I drove to the post office stopping to let my son run inside to mail a parcel. A uniformed lady suddenly appeared and said: "You've stopped on the zigzag markings. I'm giving you a ticket". I tried to explain to her that I was newly arrived in the country and did not know the significance of the zigzag markings on the road. I also mentioned that this was my birthday, thinking this might soften her determination. Handing me the ticket this keeper of British law would hear no such thing. I decided that I would take this issue to higher places, and requested trial instead of an admission of guilt and a fine. By the time I was called to traffic court it was after my car accident, so I had to enter court on crutches thinking this would ensure understanding and cancelling of the indictment. The judge listened patiently as I explained once more my status as visiting physician on sabbatical to a prestigious London institution, who had simply not understood the severe significance of the zigzag markings. Her response was immediate, crisp, and to the point – an increase in the size of the fine and penalty points for future reference. I was going to ask her if in her eyes this was a more severe offense then knocking over someone in a pedestrian crossing with a car, but my courage failed me and her honor did not seem to be one to show flexibility.

Twelve years later my knees offer various aches and pains with no particular preference for the knee involved in the accident. I reason that the regular wear and tear of aging is influencing both knees, and I'll keep doing my almost daily walks hoping they will continue to serve me. I have learnt that wearing good walking shoes together with a simple elastic bandage over the knee allows me to do my walk free of pain and discomfort. So far no further orthopaedic consultations, no imaging procedures and no intervention. Looking ahead, I am pretty sure that if in another ten years I am still alive and walking, it will be common practice to replace the knee joint for relatively mild degrees of discomfort and disability. But for the moment, I will try and manage my minor problems myself. And yes, I am particularly careful at pedestrian crossings.

THE EGG IN MY HEAD

(with thoughts on corridor consultation)

had just started a new job and the last thing I needed was another bad sinusitis attack. I walked into my ENT advisor's office just a few doors from my new office to show him some x-rays I had done over the past few years, and to ask for a prescription for a steroid nasal spray that he had previously suggested. "I have this thing on the CT which is being followed", I said lightly, handing him the latest films of my head and neck, showing a clear, round "thing" somewhere high up at the back of my throat. He studied the films, and somewhat apologetically suggested he look in my mouth. I dutifully opened my mouth as he shone the light of the scope, and I immediately saw his expression undergo a drastic change. "I'm not a big professor", he said, referring to my previous consultants, "but I must tell you that there is a mass pushing your tonsil forward. Tell me, have you been having any breathing problems?" "Well my family all tell me I snore badly these days", I offered. "You have an obstructed airway, and that "thing" will have to be operated on, soon".

The story behind the abovementioned discovery started with a problem that had been with me since the age of five. Throughout the subsequent decades I have experienced recurrent spells of common cold, followed by a feeling of hammers pounding in my forehead, and an irritating cough accompanied by days to weeks of sniffing, snorting, and coughing. I remember the endless visits to the doctor, the diagnosis of allergic sinusitis, and the tests for allergies. Looking slightly bewildered at my forearm as it was scratched and then drops of liquid applied to the scratches.

Nodding his head wisely, after he received the results, the allergist declared that I was sensitive to house dust, house pets and chocolate. As I was a fairly obedient child I was ready to stay away from dust and the dog, if necessary, but chocolate seemed unfair.

The main result of the recurrent sinusitis was the development of dependence on various inhalers I would squirt up my nostrils, a few times a day, to try and relieve the misery of the persistent cough, headaches, and sleepless nights. Overuse of the nasal spray actually resulted in increased, not decreased, sinus congestion. Later, my medical student colleagues would both mock and try to advise me as I snorted my way through lectures, bedside ward rounds, and social binges. During our short rotation in the ENT department I decided to present my problem to the resident who was teaching us. He suggested I come to his clinic and he would perform an outpatient drainage procedure. I never went, deciding like a typical medical student that the procedure would be more painful than the malady. Also, something told me even at this early stage of my training that I should exercise some caution before letting a young, relatively unexperienced resident carry out an invasive procedure on my skull. Every winter I would await the inevitable attacks, praying that the cold would not move on to a full blown episode of sinusitis, but learnt that this was the way my body behaved when invaded by a virus. I would search for the doctor, family practitioner, infectious disease specialist, or ENT surgeon who might have the answer.

I remember many cases of total misery related to this condition. The worst probably occurring during a visit to the Republic of Georgia, as a consultant for the World Bank, part of a team advising the Georgian government regarding reform of their health system.

I arrived with an established cold in the middle of winter. It was freezing cold in Tbilisi and electricity functioned only a few hours each day. Groups of secretaries in the Ministry of Health offices huddled over paraffin heaters, trying to keep warm in the cold stone building. Within hours of arriving I had started the predictable cycle of headaches, cough, and hoarseness. For two weeks I had to conduct endless interviews with people working in the health system, each interview being conducted in Georgian with simultaneous translation to English. In the evenings, I would return exhausted and miserable to my apartment where the lady of the house would send me a tray of Georgian delicacies prepared by her including borsht, an array of salads, and a huge helping of meat or other main course. She would then collect the tray after I had nibbled only a few mouthfuls, telling her daughter who knew English to ask me if I did not like her food. So in addition to feeling at death's door, I had to deal with placating the wounded ego of my landlady because of my refusal to eat her food.

Returning home, I immediately contacted an ENT specialist who had examined me frequently in the past and was familiar with my problem. At that point, in our doctor-patient relationship, it was clear that he did not have any new ideas regarding how to solve my problem. Without going through the routine of history and examination again, he said, "Let's get a CT". I always tried to be an obedient patient when seeing a doctor, and agreed.

A few days later, at nine pm, I was in the hospital's CT unit having been squeezed in as an extra patient at the end of the shift. I lay quietly as

I was moved inside the CT chamber, absorbing the new experience with interest. Within a few minutes I found myself outside the machine, pleasantly surprised at the speed of the procedure. Suddenly, the radiologist appeared next to me holding a syringe in her hand and clearly worried. "We have to inject some contrast material. You have no drug allergies, right?" I replied in the negative, and commented that I thought the examination did not require the use of contrast medium. Her worried expression increased as she mumbled "Well, even though it doesn't look serious, there's something in the para-pharyngeal area[8]". This was the moment every doctor fears, when he is told he has THE disease. The recurrent sinusitis had become the big C. My world had changed, my routine of life disappeared. I was a patient with a tumour.

After a sleepless night, I returned to my ENT colleague clutching a big brown package of CT films. He squinted at the films and the radiologist's report. "Well, it seems clearly defined, so probably there's nothing to worry about. Show it to Dr B" (the rising star in the radiology department). Dr B stared at the films during his lunch break, commenting as he lifted each film. "Very regular, not infiltrating, seems to be soft tissue." This was obviously meant to be reassuring. "So what next?" I asked deferentially. "Let's do an MRI in a few months". I was reasonably reassured. Even though no one had told me what

---

8. The space between the neck and head at the back of the mouth

was going on in this mysterious area next to the pharynx[9], the surgeon and radiologist seemed to be in agreement that there was no reason for concern.

About six months later, I dutifully reported for the MRI. This was another new experience. I was shuttled into the cavernous interior of the machine with no real preparation. The ten, maybe twenty, or thirty minutes inside were interminable. I was overwhelmed by true fear when the metallic clanging noises started to erupt around my head, and was startled by the rapid onset of claustrophobia and darkness. Every part of my body developed an itch that needed scratching, together with a feeling of total helplessness. Finding myself back in the outside world, I casually mentioned to the technician that this had been a bit of a scary experience. He smiled, "Maybe we should have given you the earphones with the music", clearly thinking to himself, *what kind of a wimp is this doctor?*

I returned to Dr B with an even bigger packet of films. He munched on his sandwich, took down some large textbooks from his bookshelves, and scoured the films. "Well, still looks regular, doesn't seem to have grown, could be a neuroma[10] or a cyst. Let's just watch it". This sounded good to me. All these words - "regular", "cyst", "neuroma" indicating that whatever it was, it was benign and I had been spared the big C.

---

9. The upper part of the digestive system also connected to the respiratory system
10. A growth or tumour of nerve tissue

Around this time I found another ENT surgeon to accompany me on my pharyngeal odyssey, a prominent recommended surgeon from a large hospital in Tel Aviv who in good collegial mode told me to come in early before he started his clinic. I duly arrived at an early hour, found his clinic, and waited patiently for his arrival. Presenting myself to him, I saw a moment of bewilderment before he remembered our phone conversation and cheerfully invited me into the kitchen at the end of the corridor. Seeing the brown folder under my arm, he immediately said "Let's have a look at those". Still standing, he proceeded to review the films against the open window. After focusing on the problem in the neck he thought for a moment then said confidently, "Whatever it is it hasn't grown over the past year. Let's watch it." After this five minute consultation I walked out of the kitchen feeling relieved, the expert's word was reassuring. I realised that like a typical doctor, I had been a little over concerned.

The next visit to a doctor was to the young specialist mentioned earlier the one who had the idea of looking inside my mouth and not just at the x-rays, and informed me that I had a large tumour in my throat. From there life had taken an unexpected turn and things moved quickly. I went home, waited for my wife to return from work, and told her to prepare for a trip overseas. I then explained that this time it would not be for pleasure, as I would be undergoing surgery for a mass in my throat. I had quickly realised two things and made a major decision. First, I had a serious problem which required surgery. Second, my problem had been misdiagnosed by serious professionals, and they were not going to be given the task of taking care of it. Within twenty-four hours I had contacted a colleague in Boston, sent the x-rays and MRI films, and a few interminable days later had a date for surgery scheduled at a prominent Boston hospital.

I had a week to kill before leaving, an awful period of worry and anger. The most evident feeling during this period was the "Why me?" phenomenon, looking at every person and asking, "Why me, why not him?" I was in serious worry mode, focusing not on whether it was or was not cancer but whether I would survive this surgery. I had never been a good student of anatomy, but I did remember the neck as a pretty tricky area with lots of nerves and glands which could be damaged during any surgical procedure. Also, I did remember our lectures in surgery, learning that any major surgery to the head and neck required an obligatory tracheotomy - opening of the airway tube, the ultimate terror of all doctors.

I tried to present a business as usual face at work and to social contacts, but my preoccupation with my body was at its highest level. I pictured myself with a paralyzed half face due to damage to a main nerve, being fed via a tube to my throat, and attached to a mobile respirator because of damage to my breathing tubes. The images of death and disability were varied and never ending. Head and neck surgery had always been associated with cancer, gross deformity, and of course death. We had laughed at it during training as only medical students and residents can. And now it was me. Why not a mild heart attack or an operable tumour in an accessible and treatable place in the abdomen?

Preparations for the trip were accompanied by a feeling of impending tragedy, not my usual state of holiday mode and eager anticipation. Eleven hours after boarding the plane we were in Boston, the white, snowy landscape doing nothing to improve my mood. My meeting with the surgeon was scheduled for the following day, the day before surgery itself.

After a jet-lagged crazy few hours' sleep I walked into the surgeon's office, a typical American doctor's office, radiating silence and efficiency. In the examination room I finally met my potential savior, a short thick-set man looking like a prototype surgeon, wearing a crisply ironed shirt, bowtie, and starched white coat with his name engraved in red on the front pocket. He was ready. He had already reviewed the medical summary and MRI films I had sent, so he proceeded to a complete medical examination including a careful look in my mouth, palpation of my neck area, and a check of my cranial nerves. He was business-like and systematic with no small talk.

On completing the examination he looked at me and asked in a puzzled voice, "What were they waiting for?" He was more puzzled then critical. He proceeded to explain that this was almost certainly a benign tumour of the parotid gland[11] which had been growing steadily, as shown by the measurements he had made on the x-rays, and was now large and causing clinical problems (mainly snoring due to some pressure on the airway). My expression asked him what happened next. "We'll give it the best shot", was his next sentence which hung in the air as I tried to understand the meaning of it. My first thought was that it was basically incurable but he would still be trying to save me. But then he proceeded to explain. "If you'd reached me a few years ago when it was still small, it would have been a relatively simple procedure. A small cut under the chin and we could have taken it out." I waited. "But now I'm not sure we can get it out that way. We might have to split the mandible and flip it up to reach the whole tumour". I tried to picture my flipped-up jawbone, while visualizing the post-operative period, with the compulsory tracheotomy.

"How long will I be with a tracheotomy?" I blurted. For the first time he smiled. "Oh we don't do THAT anymore, doctor. Just five days on an intravenous line with no food, you'll see it's not a big deal". I picked up my overnight bag and asked how to get to the ward. "You only need to arrive tomorrow morning at six am", was the cheery answer. As we were leaving, my wife decided to ask a question that had been troubling her ever since I had come

---

11. A major salivary gland

home from work and said I need surgery and it's going to be in the USA. "Tell me doctor, what will happen if he decides not to undergo surgery?" In true surgeon style, Dr R did not hesitate. "Well, he'll stop breathing". The consultation was over.

The following morning after a dream-filled night spent at the house of good friends, the taxi was waiting to drive us to the hospital. My wife and I held hands as we watched the snowy landscape through the windows of the car. The hospital was not yet awaking to its daily routine, with sleepy porters wheeling the occasional patient and cleaners vacuuming the endless corridors. We reached the operating rooms and I was shunted in immediately. An anxious nurse said, "Thank goodness, Dr R is already starting to scream at us".

I changed into my grey hospital clothes, and she measured my blood pressure. "Guess you're a little nervous", was her laconic comment at seeing the systolic blood pressure at 160 instead of my usual 120. I don't think I replied. Then a charming and alarmingly wide awake and groomed young man took my arm and within seconds slipped in an IV and taped it in perfect position. This was a simple procedure which every intern, anywhere, performs dozens of times. But his dexterity still made an impression on me. Probably because this was exactly one of those simple technical skills I never really mastered, just as I had never learnt to hammer a nail into a wall without causing plaster to crash down. He waved a little syringe and said, "You'll be a little sleepy now". And I knew this was the beginning of whatever the end to this experience. I lay back as I was wheeled into the OR itself. The smells, the white walls (maybe they were grey), the machines all familiar from my early years as student and resident, and from my own personal experiences as the patient. Then, I was lifted onto the OR table, the same charming young man sitting next to me and saying something like "See you later".

"Wake up, Basil". I was still alive. "It was amazing", said the young resident, "he took the whole thing out. Just perfect!" That sounded quite reassuring. The next time I opened my eyes I saw a young male nurse measuring my blood pressure. I was in the intermediate intensive care unit and conscious of my calves being squeezed at regular intervals, then a feeling of relaxation. Another new technology assuring no blood clots formed in my legs due to lack of movement. I dozed off again. Waking up, I now found the calf squeezing to be rather annoying. I turned to the nurse and said, "I'm awake now. I'll keep the legs moving. You can turn off the machine". His face showed no expression as he said, "That stays on till eight am tomorrow morning". I slept the night waking intermittently to the calf squeeze, and dozing off contentedly with the realisation that this was the way things are done here. This was post-operative protocol, not subject to change by any patient even if he was a knowledgeable doctor. The following morning I was walking with no real pain and suffering. Just as the surgeon had told me, it was five days on intravenous fluids only. On the morning of the sixth day I was served a soft-boiled egg and jelly, a feast to be remembered.

Two weeks later I was back home reflecting on this amazing encounter with twenty-first century technology. A pigeon egg-sized tumour had been gouged from deep in my neck, a titanium plate had been inserted between the two sides of my mandible, and apart from a long scar reaching from below my ear to under my chin I was not looking the worse for wear after the experience.

I had definitely been lucky. Firstly, it was a benign tumour. Secondly, despite the failure to make the diagnosis early on, I had reached the person with the required ability and experience to do the surgery in a hospital that provided all the necessary excellence of supportive services required for my recovery. Things were not left to chance or improvisation. From the moment I arrived for my assessment a well-oiled machine was set in motion. Including routines which allowed the surgeon to confidently say he could deal with my problem, and also tell my wife that she should wait for me in the family room and he would call when the procedure was over, about five hours after entering the operating room. And sure enough, the phone rang five hours after I parted from my wife. This was the new world of proper risk management in medicine which determined that my chances for a successful procedure depended on the expertise of the surgeon, together with a long list of lessons learnt regarding what determines a good versus a bad prognosis.

Fortunately, the poor pathway of diagnosis did not affect my outcome. Ten years later there is a fine, white zigzagging line on the left side of my neck extending to the chin as the only residue from my experience with head and neck surgery. Dr R had been very careful in our pre-surgery meeting to say that there was a small chance of recurrence of the tumour. I prefer not to think of that. I do realise that I was lucky, lucky to be born in the age of sophisticated surgery and safe anaesthesia. The addendum to this might be that the state-of-the-art technology and competent experts neutralized the potential poor results of the initial inadequate clinical management.

This episode was the first among a number of major medical issues which would affect my life in my seventh decade. I was no different from any other patient in wanting my symptoms and concerns to receive sympathetic, expert listening, and for decisions to be made with the right amount of shared participation and authoritative professional directness. Doctors learn that most medical problems connect to the adage, when you hear hoof beats, don't think of zebras, or as one of my medical school role models would say, "Common things occur commonly because they are common". But in the case of my salivary gland tumour, it indeed had been a zebra while my expert colleagues carried on for years relating to it as a horse - the animal they were used to seeing.

Medical situations are filled with stories of how an important problem was missed through poor clinical practice. Usually, meaning that first and foremost the physician had not asked the right questions or had not carried out the required routine clinical steps. In the case of my parotid tumour, this meant that from the moment the mass was discovered as an incidental finding during a CT for another purpose, it needed to be assessed and followed carefully including regular, careful measurements. In addition, there should have been regular examinations of my mouth and throat, and questions should have been asked about snoring or breathing problems. Much of clinical medical practice in any field is about routine, involving routine for mild problems, with the good clinician being on his toes thinking of the zebra when it comes by.

A TRAIN WRECK AND SALUTOGENESIS[12]

I was preparing to travel home to Be'er Sheva by train from Tel Aviv, feeling comfortable and secure after a fairly good budget meeting with the CEO of the HMO I worked for. My sense of wellbeing was accompanied by some excitement toward an upcoming trip to the USA to see my grandchildren, to be followed by a medical conference, and finally a chamber music camp in rural Vermont, a

12. Antonovsky, A. Unraveling the Mystery of Health - How People Manage Stress and Stay Well, San Francisco: Jossey-Bass Publishers, 1987

wonderful combination of professional, family, and personal activities. On arriving at the train station in Tel Aviv, I met an acquaintance with whom I chatted for a few minutes until the train pulled into the crowded station. As the crowd thronged onto the train we separated and I moved to the front carriage, settling myself in with the newspaper and assorted literature for the journey. It turned out that my acquaintance had moved towards the rear of the train. Later I would certainly regret my decision to seek solitude at the front end.

I now know that after about forty minutes, the train travelling at about 120 km/h crashed into a coal carrying truck stuck on the rails. The most frequent question after the accident had been "What do you remember from the accident?" The truth is that I remembered very little, apart from a few seconds when time stood still. I was reading the newspaper, sitting in the first carriage close to the door leading directly to the driver's compartment. I heard the shrill repetitive siren and realised that something strange was happening and then felt that my body was about to move, with no will of my own. Then, total blackness.

Later, piecing the story from my injuries, I realised I had been flung out of my seat with considerable force, through the shattered windows of the train, and then lost consciousness. This was rather fortunate as I learnt later from survivors of the accident that most of them had been thrown outside the carriage and were crying for help for at least forty-five minutes, until the first ambulances arrived. What I do remember, clearly, was opening my eyes and seeing the concerned look of a young paramedic as he informed me that I had been involved in a train accident. I remember my first reaction; I thought this must be somebody's idea of a joke. I was not the material for disasters and headlines. My mind then went very practical; I asked if my wife knew, and felt deep regret at all the time spent preparing the Beethoven quartet for my music camp that now I might not be able to attend. The paramedic took my cellular phone off my belt and asked for my wife's phone number which I was able to provide lucidly. Then, my worldly pragmatism disappeared.

I lay in a haze of semi-consciousness as the ambulance travelled to the hospital with the wailing siren constantly impinging on my sleepy state. I remember being jostled on a stretcher to the emergency room, and a vaguely familiar face of the head of the emergency room standing expectantly to receive me. My wife's face appeared and then my children at some stage, mingling with the spaceship-like atmosphere of the imaging center where my whole body was scanned. My daughter approached me and began stroking the shattered glass from my hair, my face, and my clothes.

The next few days were spent being transferred between two hospitals, shifting between foggy awareness, restless sleep in intensive care units, and lying in ambulances with sirens screaming. Faces of my wife and children, nurses, doctors and orderlies blurred in front of me with the vague memory of being funneled into a CT chamber, but no memory remaining of the move to the operating room where my crushed third vertebra in my neck was removed, a bone graft inserted, and a titanium plate placed to fixate my spine. Trying to stay awake and communicate with my family who seemed to have some concern in their expressions, I remember wondering why I was covered in glass fragments. I do recall though, vividly, looking up at a baby faced figure in a leather motorcycle jacket standing next to me who introduced himself as the surgeon who would be fixing my broken neck, including my comment that he should finish high school first.

Following surgery, I was in the surgical intensive care unit until my condition stabilized and then transferred to a regular ward. This posed a dilemma for those responsible. Clearly, I was an orthopaedic case. A vertebral bone in my neck had been broken but I had also experienced damage to my spine, had clear neurologic damage to my right arm, and had multiple trauma and some fractures in many parts of my body. I had also lost consciousness after a probable blow to the head, a clearly neurologic problem.

Medicine today demands pigeonholing - one can be a neurology, cardiology, or gastroenterology case, each ward finding reasons to jealously guard the few, if any, remaining beds available for new patients. And so, even in the sprawling, ivory tower hospital which housed all the modern glories of medical advances I was some kind of orphan. Finally, a decision was made to place me in a general surgery ward. I assume not through a positive decision that this was an appropriate place to take care of the patient with multiple surgical and medical issues, but rather a negative decision that other departments either had no bed available, or simply did not want a patient with multiple trauma to be admitted.

In the general surgery ward, a young blonde resident with a computer stood by my side asking the rote questions required by the medical history. Staring at her computer screen, balanced on a trolley, she failed to make any eye contact with me. She was clearly bewildered. I was not a case for gastrectomy - removal of the stomach, or colectomy - removal of the colon, or removal of any other portion of the human body. A case of head trauma, fractured neck vertebra, multiple rib fractures, and bruising of the entire body was clearly not a general surgery issue.

The horizontal doctor was now totally dependent on his environment to take care of all his basic needs. Reality was setting in. I realised I would not be travelling to the USA in a week's time, pain was starting to occupy most places in my body, and I was feeling very uncomfortable with my head encased in a hard collar digging into the back of my head. Moving was difficult, eating was difficult, performing bodily functions was difficult, and making polite conversation was exhausting as family and friends appeared at my side continuously.

Then, a psychologist colleague who was visiting me remarked, "What you really need now is some salutogenesis". Even in my confused state I was able to recall the late Aaron Antonowsky, the medical sociologist, who had been my next-door neighbour for many years in Be'er Sheva. Aaron was a medical sociologist of considerable repute. He joined the faculty of the new medical school, stressing a major shift in medical education and educating towards the community, as opposed to the hospital, as the key target. He had preached both students and faculty incessantly with his theory of salutogenesis, basically describing how some people managed to stay well even when severely stressed. One of his theory keys was related to what he called one's Sense of Coherence, involving three elements: *comprehensibility* - a sense that you understand events in your life, *manageability* - that you have the tools to control events, and *meaningfulness* - basically that one can believe that life is worth living. I confess that as a new young faculty member I was not always very sympathetic to the constant reminder from Aaron, asking at every discussion about a patient or medical problem, "Why don't you ask people how they stay well instead of asking why they are sick?" At the time, it did not seem very relevant to me. But now, from the horizontal position I was in, it slowly dawned on me that what I needed most was some Sense of Coherence. I needed to understand what had happened and get an idea about the future. I needed to recruit all my tools and resources to deal with the event, and I also had to believe that it was worth all the effort.

From this moment it became almost a question of me versus my environment. The surgery was technically successful, but my right arm was paralyzed with significant neurological loss in other areas. I had bruises from my scalp down to my toes, and a few fractured ribs witness to the force I was thrown from my seat during the accident. Pain was everywhere. Nausea accompanied the smell or even talk of food that together with severe constipation, and exhaustion, I was not feeling very positive regarding my life. And, the hospital environment was of no help to any sense of coherence. After years of walking from bed to bed on ward rounds in hospitals, I now saw first-hand from my new vantage point that the hospital environment was basically directed at the doctors and nurses, while the patient was mostly an observer and expected to be a passive one.

There was clear concern regarding the paralysis of my right arm. The discussion between various consultants was whether this was due to the spinal injury, or caused by damage to the brachial plexus - the bundle of nerves found between the shoulder and arm. I strained to interpret muttered comments and elements of body language as the knowledgeable consultants discussed my case on ward rounds. As function returned to the arm it was decided that my main injury was indeed to the cervical spinal cord, and the slow process of rehabilitation began.

I had been moved from the main hospital to the

rehabilitation ward in order to start using my body again with the help of a team of specialists including physical therapists, occupational therapists, and the occasional psychologist or social worker to attend to my disturbed psyche.

Following my arrival in the rehabilitation ward, a nurse speedily arrived with a wheelchair and informed me in an authoritative tone that this was how I was to move from now on. Now that I had understood my problem, I had to deal with the manageability part of Antonovsky's salutogenesis. This involved dealing with a host of practical issues. There was a need to learn wheelchair mobility, mainly using my legs as my arms were not yet very functional. Things I had always taken completely for granted, such as getting up from the lying position in bed and going to the bathroom, had now become major life challenges.

The senior medical director in the HMO was now focusing on turning to the left side, bending the knees, rolling off the bed, and then moving into a wheelchair. My world had contracted, my body now center stage. Satisfaction now involved a successful trip to the bathroom or the physical therapy room, instead of passing a budget at a meeting or solving the lack of a paediatrician in one of the towns in the area.

The Philadelphia collar around my neck was probably the item that had saved my life, and should therefore have been treated with honor and thanks. But it was extremely uncomfortable to have your head connected to your body by an apparatus equivalent to some piece of medieval armor, though made out of plastic, which enabled lying only on the back and making it impossible to turn the head. I began to experience fairly severe pain at the back of the head, at the exact point where the collar touched the scalp area. When I began to repeatedly mention that it was moving from discomfort to real pain the staff hastened to explain that, "Yes, the collar is very uncomfortable, but you'll get used to it". This was one in many other occasions I would learn that the medical staff wants to hear things that are familiar and manageable from the patient, and that any perceived exaggeration of feelings or symptoms require an authoritative firm answer, leaving no place for further discussion.

By the time my persistent nagging had increased to unpleasant levels the damage was done. A nasty pressure sore had developed at the site. I thought back to one of my first clinical teachers in medical school who never failed to remind his residents, "Listen to the patient". I had seen pressure sores many times in my medical career. A phenomenon associated in my mind with old, semi-conscious patients in nursing homes who were unable to move without help, and if were not actively turned over regularly developed painful sores where the body was in contact with a hard surface.

The sore at the back of my scalp rapidly developed into a bag of smelly pus and was certainly a reminder of how much suffering in hospitals is due to preventable problems. Iatrogenic problems - caused by the treatment process - are today a part of every doctor's experience, whether due to administration of wrong medication or a mistaken action in surgery. Numerous articles in medical literature attest to the costs iatrogenic problems have in terms of money and suffering to the patient and system. This pressure sore should not have happened and could have easily been prevented if someone had taken notice when I said "It really hurts!" Fortunately, this pressure sore on my scalp was not in my range of vision, I could only smell it. I understood from the reactions of my family members who witnessed the change of bandage or removal of dead skin, by one of the staff, that it was not a pleasant sight.

Still, the ultimate insult from this hospital-induced problem occurred one morning when I was sitting in my wheelchair in my room, looking out of the window. I heard the familiar footsteps of the chief nurse coming down the corridor, and then heard her voice clearly talking to the person she was accompanying. The next thing was feeling excruciating pain in my scalp followed by a male voice saying, "That's fine, we'll see it again next week", followed by the sounds of footsteps moving away from the room. I turned the wheelchair around but there was no one to be seen. I wheeled myself to the nurses' station and asked the chief nurse, "Who just visited me in my room?" She smiled and said that this was the consultant plastic surgeon. I was in shock. I knew that many physicians were lacking in empathy and even in basic communication skills. But somehow, the thought that a doctor could enter a patient's room as a consultant and complete his task without even attempting to look the patient in the eye, or say, "Good morning, I am Dr…," was an epiphany. An indication of how low the art of clinical medicine could go.

As the days passed by, I started to relate to the simple day-to-day functioning of my body. I now had to deal with bodily functions that up to now had been taken for granted. The taking in of food and its elimination became prime issues to deal with - my appetite had disappeared. For someone who had always enjoyed food as one of life's more enjoyable pastimes, finding myself not only uninterested but even repelled by the thought of any kind of food was a novel and unpleasant phenomenon. I dreaded the smell of the food trays as they arrived for the lunchtime meal usually immediately following breakfast and the attempts, that remained unresponsive, to force me to eat protein supplements or my wife's chicken soup. I knew my body needed nutrition, and much more than usual, as it tried to adapt to the trauma sustained in the train crash and the subsequent surgery. But the extreme appetite loss together with the constipation tested me beyond my poor neurologic function. Each day I swallowed more laxatives of increasing potency and felt my colon expand with no sign that anything was going to exit from down below.

As I watched my body shed seventeen kilograms

from its normal healthy eighty kilograms, I could only reflect on the irony of the efforts I had made, from time to time, to lose five kilos compared with this effortless descent to true skinniness. Food became an enemy, the smell of lunchtime chicken or schnitzel were enough to cause my stomach to heave with refusal. The manageability part of my sense of coherence was no easy task.

The basics of everyday life, from moving around to eating to eliminating, were now all major life challenges. Yet, the third element of my sense of coherence, the belief that what happens is worth caring about, was the most difficult. My apparent normal intellectual function, including my ability to joke my way through most situations seemed to indicate that my brain was OK. I cheerily answered the question "How are you today?" with the answer, "Better than yesterday and not as good as tomorrow". I had always been a people-pleasing type, so it was quite in character for me to be chirpily convincing to my medical team that all was going well. No bad dreams, no memories of the event, and my smiling responses indicated to the treatment team that I had no PTSD - Post Traumatic Stress Disorder. My initial hospital discharge did list "R/O TBI", a typical doctors' incomprehensible jargon, which basically said Rule Out Traumatic Brain Injury.

I reflected on this frequently over the years, and decided that it should have been reasonable to assume that somebody who had lost consciousness for nearly an hour, after having his body flung from a train impacting at high speed would most probably have had some degree of TBI. I realised that my brain had certainly actively participated in my trauma. I did not read anything other than headlines of a newspaper, nor listened to music for at least a year after the event. This together with an inability to concentrate on any topic for more than ten minutes, a marked increase in irritability, and periods of wondering whether it was worth caring about the future that translates as depression, all indicated that I had indeed suffered brain injury even if it was far less visible than the spinal insult.

Re·ha·bil·i·ta·tion - the action or process of rehabilitating or of being rehabilitated, **A:** the *physical* restoration of a sick or disabled person by therapeutic measures and reeducation to participation **in the activities of a normal life** within the limitations of the person's physical disability **B:** the process of restoring an individual to a useful and constructive place **in society** especially through some form of vocational, correctional, or therapeutic retraining[13]. I only read this definition of rehabilitation sometime after going through the process and found it very helpful not only as a theoretical definition of a process, but also as a guideline for where I needed to go. I needed to physically restore myself to participation in the activities of normal life. To those normal activities that normal people never think twice about, now

13. Merriam Webster Dictionary, Revised April 2016, Encyclopedia Britannica

so central to my daily coherence and being. I also needed to be restored to a useful and constructive place in society. Would this be as a health services manager, a school patrol officer, or perhaps as an early retired physician to sit on a committee for granting disability rights? At the time when I could not move, eat, or write independently the ultimate scenario was unclear.

The period in full-time rehabilitation provided much time to reflect on my situation regarding the others in my world. I was handicapped and very much aware of my dependence on people and appliances to cope with life. I looked with envy at people walking out of the building, or at the staff doing their regular chores. Using their arms and legs without having to think about the function they were performing while I had difficulty moving food from the spoon to my mouth, moving in and out of bed, and toilet issues were major challenges. But as I slowly regained function and watched the quadriplegic patients struggle with breathing and responding to human contact, or the young victims of car accidents struggling to ambulate with their paralyzed legs I realised how privileged I was. I realised that I was improving every day. Slowly returning to being able to shower alone, shave myself, and eat with some degree of social finesse. I saw how the severely paralyzed returned day after day to their therapists, battling to achieve some tiny degree of progress. I slowly had to shake off the role of the doctor badly injured in the train accident, as I became one of the denizens of the rehabilitation ward requiring less and less help and moving toward discharge to the regular world.

After two months of full-time hospitalisation, I was sent home to continue part time therapy as an ambulatory patient. Once more, a word that suddenly had new meaning for me. An ambulatory patient indicated that I had graduated from being a horizontal dependent patient to one who can ambulate, i.e. get around independently. But I had certainly not fulfilled the definition of rehabilitation. I was not yet physically restored and I had certainly not taken my place back in society. I was slowly weaned from formal physical and occupational therapy - the physical therapists dealing with the body and legs, the occupational therapists with the arms, as I strengthened my body and slowly regained function.

I still could not do many movements with my right arm; my writing was terrible and I was still suffering from a lot of pain. I was also afraid of the responsibility of looking after my body without a team to support me and a strict daily routine of treatments. I felt I was not ready to control my own time. Nonetheless, and although I would have preferred someone else to do the job, six months after the accident I found myself taking on the role of patient manager. I had a family practitioner, a competent and empathetic physician who knew me well through many of my past medical experiences. But I knew I could not expect her to understand my needs, and where to find answers to the questions I had. I assumed that she too had not learnt much about rehabilitation at medical school and in her practice had encountered few, if any, patients with diagnoses of a spinal injury and possible brain injury.

So where was I at this point? I was physically markedly improved. I could use both arms and legs reasonably well, though most of the time my right shoulder was positioned somewhere approaching the level of my chin with my head tilted toward the same side. I was also coping with constant pain in my right arm which was partly responsible for the poor positioning of my shoulder and head. At this point, I became exposed to a long list of people who wished to offer advice regarding my problems. Most of them knew someone who "had just the same problem", and had gone to a particular therapist who had literally "saved their life". Slowly, I returned to my job as a health services manager and child development consultant, taking regular long walks in the park, with my wife quietly giving me the message that it was business as usual. I read avidly, savored every moment spent with my grandchildren and felt that, yes, it had been worth it all.

Still, I received constant reminders that though my condition had improved to almost normal levels, I was far from normal. When demonstrating to children in my clinic how I wanted them to stand on one leg for a few seconds, I had to perform this act on the left leg only. Trying this on the right leg would have me stumbling and falling to the floor. I was also tired and needed an afternoon nap to restore my brain's ability to think clearly.

A key part of my rehabilitation process was

my return to playing chamber music. Music had always been an important part of my life, enjoying playing in various groups, mainly string quartets. I was a fairly good first violinist. I was able to play and lead groups playing most of the music written by the giants of chamber music Haydn, Mozart, Beethoven, Brahms and more.

In the early days following my accident, with a totally paralyzed right arm, I began to prepare myself for a future without playing music. I had serious conversations with myself. Convincing myself that I have had many happy years of playing music and that it was now the time to be a good listener. A cellist colleague visited me during my rehabilitation period in hospital and reminded me how she had returned to playing after a mild stroke, urging me not to give up hope of playing again. On returning home, she contacted me and said she had organized a string quartet and I was to play second violin. I agreed to give it a try and duly arrived at the appointed time, launching into a string quartet of Haydn. I ached everywhere. Holding the instrument under my chin was torture. And the sound, the sound! Screeching at the level of a violin beginner was the only way to describe the experience. My fingers responded poorly, I missed most of the right notes, and half way through the quartet I raised the white flag. This part of my life was not going to return, I thought.

Some months later, a physician-cum-violinist colleague suggested we try to play some violin duets. I hesitantly agreed. We proceeded to play a simple duet, and to my surprise there was a change. I could master my fingers of my left hand better, my right arm could move the bow, and the sound was almost tolerable. I was encouraged and began to add some music to my daily routine. At first things moved slowly. The playing of pieces I knew well still presenting a major challenge. But then, fairly suddenly, I felt a leap forward and increasing proficiency in my playing. I was not playing with the same technical ability I had before the accident, but I was rapidly reaching an ability to play in a group again.

Fortunately some years prior to the accident I had started playing the viola, the violin's bigger brother. I now found that the instrument was a little easier to manage than the violin and was soon playing chamber music again, mainly as a violist with proficiency pretty close to my previous level. This return to playing music astonished me. After six months of dealing with an almost useless and very painful right arm, extreme weakness in both arms, and a very befuddled brain, here I was dealing with the complexities of chamber music playing, almost as if there had been no intervening accident damaging my brain and spinal cord. I read the notes in the alto key, something that had always challenged me in the past. I remembered the slight difference in the positioning of the fingers on the viola, compared with the violin, and marveled how my damaged right arm resumed the ability to move the bow over the strings.

I realised that I was demonstrating an important part of scientific knowledge regarding the human brain, the phenomenon of plasticity. The ability of the brain to bounce back from trauma and regain lost functions. It was clear that there had been major activity in my brain since it struck the wall of the train carriage as I was thrown out of my seat on impact. Somehow, some damaged nerves and nerve connections had re-organized allowing me to remember past learning regarding playing the violin, while others were now granting me the technical ability to play once again. This was an exciting realization. Not only because it allowed me to appreciate my return to active participation in music, but also it was living proof that nerve damage was not irreversible and that even a sixty-year-old could regain lost function.

I feel I have been very lucky. Firstly because another few millimeters of trauma to my neck and I would either have been quadriplegic or dead. Secondly, I was clearly managed well at the site of the accident and in surgery. Thirdly, I have a rich supportive environment of family and friends. I still have ongoing neuropathic pain in my right arm with hypersensitivity to touch over a small area of my upper arm, making the touch of a sleeve a painful experience. But I am here! Living a full life and awake every morning thinking of the less fortunate ones. Those with no ability to perform most of life's functions alone and who would be dependent on people and technology to keep them functioning for the rest of their lives, their future harsh and gloomy. Also, I think of how my old neighbour Antonowsky must look down on me from heaven and say, "I told you so".

DOCTOR IT HURTS

Wearing a shirt with sleeves has always been taken for granted. Not something I would ever think would be of any significance regarding the quality of my life. Today my wardrobe is full of various sleeveless garments, from the simple vest to keep warm in the winter to a range of models belonging to the sport super stars, of different colours and materials. Waiting patiently for me to return from work or a social outing, these are now worn throughout the year. First thing I do when I come home is tear off the long sleeve garment and breathe out a long sigh of relief, as the sleeveless shirt is donned. And if I should bump into the occasional acquaintance during my power walk in the park, who with a puzzled look will ask, "Aren't you cold?" I no longer have the patience to start with the explanation. So just a big smile as I say, "No", and march on. I have neuropathic pain with allodynia - pain from stimuli which are not normally painful. Practically, the lightest touch to my right upper arm feels like being stroked with barbed wire.

Following the train accident, most of the pain I experienced was rather predictable. Bruises can hurt especially when in areas close to bone such as on the tibia[14], the arms, or the skull. Fractured ribs are notorious for severe pain with little to do about it. There were also pains around the entire right shoulder area which had suffered a severe direct blow.

Shortly after surgery (involving removal of the fractured vertebra, insertion of a bone graft, and fixation of the cervical spine with a titanium plate), a doctor and nurse approached me and introduced themselves as The Pain Team. They said I had a morphine syringe next to me, and I could initiate a pulse of painkilling morphine into my vein whenever it felt necessary. "Use the morphine freely, don't wait for the pain to get bad. There's no need to suffer." Even though the pain was not too severe at this stage, this was reassuring. Dutifully monitoring my pain, I gave the occasional push on the syringe as instructed. The nurses approached me on every shift and would ask, "On a scale of one

14. Shinbone

to ten, how bad is the pain?" At first the answer was quite easy. The pain not being bad, I could offer a cheerful two or three. But around the third post-surgery day things became more complicated. I became more conscious of pain in the region of my neck and back which I attributed to having to spend twenty-four hours with the hard, uncomfortable Philadelphia collar around my neck. The collar limited movement of my head and the attached body as various areas of my back and neck went into muscle spasm. My ribs ached and there was also dull pain from the numerous bruises. So now when the nurses popped the question "How bad is the pain?" I had a problem. The neck was a six on the pain scale, the back around four, the ribs a definite seven and the bruises another six. Should I offer all the numbers? Or should I add them up and give an average? Or just give the number for the worst pain? The first time I presented my dilemma to the nurse she looked at me a little bewildered and said, "Just give a number". So she got an average. This left me wondering what would this do to the ward statistics regarding pain management, or to the paper that maybe one of the doctors would want to write.

Meanwhile, the pain team appeared every few days to ask how I was coping. After a few days the morphine self-regulating pump had come out of my vein in the middle of the night, and I said there was no need to re-insert it. The pain team seemed a bit peeved, but agreed to go along with me on a more conservative regime. Oral drugs were prescribed on a fixed regime, from the milder to the stronger, till the pains gradually receded. Then, I slowly became aware of the new pain.

Casual attire, t-shirts and shorts, was the dress rule in the rehabilitation ward. The short sleeve of my cotton t-shirts began to irritate my upper right arm, to the extent I had to roll the sleeve over my shoulder to decrease contact with the skin. I asked the nurses for an elastic bandage to wrap around my upper arm to neutralize this new irritation. This was followed by a dull inner pain in the arm sometimes accompanied by a feeling of warm oil oozing under my skin. I mentioned these new puzzling phenomena to the doctors on the main weekly ward round, and saw a smile of wisdom with some condescension cross their faces. The term *Neuropathic pain* was mentioned for the first time in this hospitalisation, and I must confess in my medical career as well. Little did I know that the limiting factor to a normal life had arrived.

The first thing I learnt about this new passenger in my body was that it did not play by the rules. The usual pain medications did not do anything, and I was to start on a path of personal pharmacology that was complex, poorly understood, and most importantly did not seem to work very well. Some drugs caused side effects before any significant improvement in the pain was felt. As a physician I knew that the term side effects had usually meant what the manufacturers were obliged to write in the paper inside the box of pills. Now, I was experiencing them all - sleepiness, dizziness, wild dreams, constipation, you name it. And the most interesting and maddening aspect of neuropathic pain is its heterogeneity and obstinacy. It is not a single type of symptom, not a toothache that progresses from a mild ache to unbearable torment with a more or less predictable reaction to a progressively aggressive drug regime. Instead, I experienced a wide range of phenomena related to the umbrella of neuropathic pain progressing throughout the day.

On waking up the pain was usually mild, a feeling of discomfort in the upper arm. On moving out of bed the feeling of warm oil or scratching under the skin began, some days mild and on other days more severe. The allodynia - the exquisite sensitivity of a small area over my right upper arm, measured out by various experts to the last millimeter, appeared as I pulled on a shirt. The slightest touch to that area registered as a searing shriek of pain in my brain. Then a dull, underlying pain developed its crescendo towards the evening, followed by totally unpredictable electric shocks shooting into the shoulder area, and resulting in a twitch of the arm and wincing of the face. The climax of the day, the final ingredient of the pain soup was a feeling of a heavy weight pushing down on the shoulder before I threw off the shirt and flopped on the bed, lying still, and enjoying the blessed freedom from my pain partner. Yes, at least rest calmed the pain demons.

Prior to my initiation into the world of chronic pain, my conception of pain and pain management had been fairly traditional. Pain was an unpleasant sensation accompanying trauma or illness, a cut or influenza, which various local creams or pills could relieve. Both as a patient and as physician I could admire the new technologies like the self-regulated morphine IV following surgery, as well as the amazing ability of the brain to use its own chemicals through hypnosis to conquer pain. The comforting knowledge was that there is always another step to take that would end the pain. But my neuropathic devil defied the rules. The chemical pathway of various drugs alone and then in combination, the nerve stimulation, acupuncture, and spinal injections all failed to affect the daily cycle of mild to moderate to severe pain.

Slowly, I sensed the need for a paradigm shift from "Stopping the pain" to "Living with the pain". Making this shift has been a gradual process. Only after meeting many neurologists and pain gurus did the need for this change in attitude dawn on me. The first time my question, "When will this pain go away?" was answered with "Well, we don't really know", I was seized by a minor panic attack. Up to now, the pain was another symptom like sleepiness or constipation which had to be endured, but had in my mind a finite point; some future morning I would awake, smile, and say, "It's gone". Now, I was being told about something that might last weeks, months, years, or might never disappear. Could I really carry on with life as the flames of hell constantly licked my arms? Could I tattoo a message on my right upper arm, or have all my shirts engraved with giant letters "DO NOT TOUCH"?

I mulled over the many people living with chronic illness, monitoring heart disease or diabetes. One can forget about blood sugar or cholesterol while at work or play, but how does one forget pain? As the panic subsided I took the first healing step; accept pain as my co-traveler, still to be fought if possible but more importantly to be accepted and managed as part of the whole life experience.

As with most medical problems, there is always the possibility of a second opinion. Something I have always strongly believed in and encouraged people to do before undergoing surgery, or jumping off a building in despair because of their problem. My specialist consultation regarding pain began during my hospitalisation following the train accident and the long period in rehabilitation. As soon as neuropathic pain was diagnosed, I was sent to see one of the doctors working in the rehabilitation unit who was said to be an expert in the field. He was a serious American-trained specialist who listened attentively and examined me thoroughly. He suggested trying to define the area of high pain sensitivity in the arm and proceeded to touch my arm with a needle. Starting far away from the tender area he slowly moved inwards to the point I screamed and threw my arm up in the air. He mapped out an area of about one square centimeter as the place responsible for my suffering. Ten years later, this patch of skin still does not allow the lightest touch of a shirt sleeve or a friendly tap, my brain interpreting these as excruciating pain. Despite the interest and efforts to adjust medication the pain continued.

I travelled to the USA and consulted with a pain specialist at a leading New England hospital. She suggested I return to a specialist in Israel who had trained with her. A pain specialist in London listened carefully and examined me. Expressing interest in the intensity of pain when my right upper arm was touched, I agreed to have the level of pain measured in his laboratory. Sure enough, the pain intensity hit the top of the scale. Back home, I was referred to a rising star in the pain field. He listened to my story and assured me things would improve if I would make some medication adjustments. Slowly it was dawning on me that none of these pain experts were really able to do anything dramatic, and I was once more coming to terms with the reality that I was going to be living with neuropathic pain for a long time.

By this time I had noticed some strange aspects of the pain. Firstly, from the early stages of rehabilitation it became clear to me that the moment I lay on the bed, even before falling asleep, the pain was gone. The creeping spiders and boiling oil under my skin, the heavy load on my shoulders, and the single point drill in my arm all miraculously disappeared as my body sank into the pillows and mattress. Secondly, absorption in work, a movie, a book, or a conversation, seemed to temporarily drive the pain into the back seat. On returning to part-time work after completing my formal rehabilitation program, I would wait for a ride to work with one of the secretaries. I would climb into the car slowly, gritting my teeth and mumbling a reply to the cheery "good morning" greeting and sat hunched up cursing myself for agreeing to go back to work. I then walked into my office, started looking at some papers, made some telephone calls and the pain was forgotten till the end of the day when I returned home. It became clear to me that the pain story was more complicated then I had previously thought, or had been taught.

I regularly visited a pain specialist. She was an attentive, sensitive physician. Just meeting with her empathetic manner was therapeutic. After a few visits she happily informed me that I was an eligible candidate for medical cannabis therapy. My ears pricked up. I had only tried smoking pot once or twice in my life, and remembered that I had not undergone a major change of state during those experiences. Maybe a little happier, maybe enjoying listening to a Beethoven quartet with some heightening of emotion, but that was it. Nonetheless, it seemed worth a try.

I received my formal certificate of eligibility for cannabis therapy from the Ministry of Health and was pleased to see that the official provider was a few minutes' walk from my apartment. I entered the inconspicuous apartment and was welcomed by a young man who recorded my history and asked if I knew how to smoke the weed. I was then seated on a couch in a room where a number of youngish people were sitting and smoking with gusto. My host lit my joint and I proceeded to begin inhaling alongside my new peer group. My immediate partner on the couch was busy rolling joints and suggested I do the same. As this seemed to be the way time was spent during "therapy", I readily agreed and started trying to roll my first joint. Somehow, what seemed so easy when demonstrated by my experienced neighbour was an unsurmountable technical challenge for me. Shreds of the precious weed fell all over the couch and onto the floor. I was unable to seal the paper to create a reasonable looking joint and realised that as much as I had been technically inept in the past, three months post neck injury, my finger coordination now was effectively zero. Fortunately, my partner who was patient and understanding helped me roll at least one decent joint to show my host, and I was sent home with a box of ready rolled smokes to continue twice daily.

Alas, after pouring over the literature and seeing that it indeed did hold out hope for me, and despite my enthusiasm for this new field of therapy it was not to be. I would light my joint next to my bedroom window, inhale the pungent fumes, and try to exhale through the window. But regardless how hard I tried, the room absorbed the smell and my clothes and bed linens all stank of weed smoke. My mouth felt like a birdcage and I needed to sleep. No euphoria and no real change in pain. My pain doctor urged me not to give up so I returned a few more times to try purer types of marijuana, and even a pure extract in powder form. To the great surprise of some of my marijuana attached friends I did not become a fellow traveler, even after being assured that the stuff I was getting was of the highest quality…

Years later, the partnership continues. My neuropathic pain has not been defeated completely, but has definitely decreased progressively over the years. However, there are still bad days and good days which are difficult to predict. Very hot and dry days do seem to set off the electricity in the arms. On other days I find myself progressively aware of pain in both my arms, accompanied by terrific sensitivity to touch, tiredness, and irritability beyond the normal range. I know now that these are the days when I must turn off the inputs from the surrounding world as early as possible. I get into bed early, take a small dose of a sleeping pill, and know that I will wake up the next morning refreshed and without pain. Also, tiredness, boredom, or emotional tension send the pain factor soaring.

I have tried to understand the complexity of neuropathic pain in the medical literature; the interaction of perceived pain at the skin level, the damaged peripheral nerves and spinal cord roots, and the ultimate perception of pain within the brain.

I have discovered that life can be lived in parallel with neuropathic pain. I dress every morning, go to work and do all the things that working people, even physician managers do - meetings, writing documents, talking on the phone, and overseas travel. I try to be a functional spouse, parent, and grandfather. People stopped asking me how I feel, and I no longer have the need to describe my sorry post-trauma state to everyone I meet. I try to advise and help my friends who are starting to meet a range of illness and disability related to our age and stage. I stopped opening my eyes every morning with the first thought that *Perhaps it's gone?* The complex phenomenon of neuropathic pain became part of my being. Less a challenger, more a fellow traveler to be tolerated not dismissed.

The pain journey is an ongoing part of my experience with major trauma. The bruises have vanished, the neck now functions fairly well, and my ageing body seems to serve me as much as that of my friends and colleagues. I still take pain medication every morning and evening, and visit a pain specialist a few times a year. I have not taken the ultimate test of stopping the medications to see if I can function without them. Partly this stems from fear of worsening of the pain that I have become accustomed to, and partly from some belief that these pills I swallow are important and indeed calm the damaged nerves and help me maintain normal function. I have tried lowering the dose of the various medications, from time to time, and it seems I have reached a level of minimal dosage below which the pain becomes worse.

A major lesson regarding pain has been the understanding that much of the pain relates to the perception of that pain. In my specific case, I learnt early during my slow rehabilitation from the spinal injury that pain did not only cease after taking a pill, but also, as previously mentioned, it could be moved into the background. An hour after immersing myself in the work on my desk, sitting in a meeting, or addressing issues of other people's medical problems, when playing with my grandchildren, reading a good book, playing a string quartet, or enjoying a meal with friends the pain was forgotten. Distraction was crucial.

Perhaps this was for me the meaning of the encouraging phrase, "Don't lose hope". Maybe hope really meant giving a signal to the damaged nervous system not to give up, and to re-organize for the continuation of life. And even if some pain is there I could learn to live with it, like a difficult neighbour or a bad day at the office. I know there are many people in this world who live with pain far worse than mine, some of them continuously looking for a new pill, a new refinement of marijuana, or a new fancy technology to relieve their misery. Others have found the way to accept the pain as part of their existence, and degrade its importance so they can enjoy everything else in life.

Chronic pain is not visible like paraplegia or Parkinson's disease. I look quite normal though sometimes I feel that maybe it would be preferable for my pain level to show as a red blotch on the skin, or contortion of the limbs so that people would understand that today is a bad day; a day with some suffering, a day where it is difficult for me to concentrate, a day where I prefer not to be talking to people. Every morning I try to remind myself that I was a few millimeters from being a quadriplegic, and that basically I have a well-functioning body which tries to keep up the recommended levels of physical activity. Perhaps, pain now part of my being, it is a life challenge meant to teach me that the human body can deal with practically anything, even the most unpleasant and complex of incurable sensations. And this has been the ultimate lesson for me regarding the commonest of complaints, "Doctor, it hurts!"

LOSING MY SENSES

There are many things we take for granted regarding our bodies. We expect our hearts to beat, to be able to breathe in and out, and that our muscles will function properly to allow us to walk, talk, eat, and interact as needed. We also need to smell the roast chicken being prepared for dinner, to hear the softest plucking of the harp strings in the concert hall, or see the first steps of a child. Like so many other things in life, we only appreciate these abilities when we start to lose them.

My ears were the first to signal that not all was right. My wife had been indicating to me for some considerable time that even though she was sure that a lot of my non-responding to her voice was passive-aggressive behavior, related to not wanting to respond, i.e. "Have you taken care of the problem with the phone? Have you found a dermatologist for your daughter?", at least some of the time I was not hearing well. I also noticed that in some specific situations such as casual dinner conversations or watching a play I was missing a lot. I finally agreed to go for a hearing test. I duly sat in the soundproof booth while the audiologist sent sounds and words through to my earphones from the adjacent room. I found it a bit tricky to hear when she deliberately overshadowed the sounds with a background of swishing water, but was still confident that I had responded correctly to most sounds and therefore had minimal, if any, hearing loss. My confidence was swiftly drained when the examination results showed clear loss of hearing in both ears.

The cause was most probably related to an event that occurred during my period of training as a doctor in the Israeli army. During my officers' course I was present at a tank division shooting range. I remember taking the first aid kit and relaxing with a book a few hundred meters away from the monstrous tanks, lining up for the practice session. As with most such events in the military the preparation took forever with officious officers running around and shouting orders to each other, while the bored-looking soldiers performed the minimal required rituals to prepare the tanks for the event. My peaceful reverie was suddenly disturbed by a sound that was not so much heard but felt. BOOM does not really describe the noise accompanying shells discharged from a tank's artillery. The BOOM, WHAM, SHAZAM shook my body and were followed by a chorus of bells ringing and tingling in my ears as all other sounds were put on hold. The tingling was not momentary and had worried me for a considerable period after the event, but then disappeared and was forgotten.

Now, some thirty years later, I was looking at the maze of symbols and numbers showing the results of the hearing test while being told that this was a classic picture of damage to the hair cells of the sensitive part of the inner ear, most probably directly related to that single blast from the Patton tank cannons. Today, nobody is in the vicinity of the firing artillery shells without the use of large ear coverings, blocking and protecting the inner ear from receiving the knockout blow to its most sensitive parts.

Having at least received some vindication for my years of "not listening", the time had come to seek a solution for the problem. The audiologist said I certainly needed hearing aids and proceeded to present the various alternatives. At this point ego preservation crept in. Even though well in my sixties, I was not ready for that step of putting a prominent bulge onto my spectacle frames which would clearly mark me as an old codger. I therefore opted for a sleek, inconspicuous model that hid behind the earlobe and could be ordered in a colour to match the hair or skin. The appliance arrived and I was invited back to be trained how to use it. I was immediately amazed by the noise of the air conditioner sounding like a Boeing 747 landing in the room. Also, there was no doubt I was hearing the spoken voice much more clearly. I felt I was about to become a much more sociable character than I had been in the last few years.

Together with the training regarding how to use the little machines I was also drilled regarding how to maintain them. The first step was to know how to replace the batteries when needed. The "when needed" proved to be a much shorter period of time than I thought, and highly unpredictable. The brilliant little machine would send a long blast of sound like a trumpet fanfare to warn that in about ten minutes time the battery charge would be depleted. Replacing the battery was a simple act of opening the earpiece behind the earlobe, discharging the old battery, and inserting the new one as shown on the diagram inside. While this sounded like a simple procedure, it took quite a few tries for me to master the extraction of the tiny battery from its little compartment, open and discharge a new battery from the battery pack, and successfully insert it into the correct position. Clearly, I was never required to change the batteries for both machines at the same time, so I had to be sure that extra batteries were always at hand in the pockets of a jacket or trousers. This was to prove to be the easy part of hearing aid maintenance.

The other part of maintenance involved cleaning

the small receiver seated in a molded plastic model of the canal that fitted into the ear. This was tricky because I produced large amounts of ear wax (apparently, there are heavy and light ear wax producers). I was given a set of toothpick-like cleaners and was expected to regularly flip out a tiny disposable lining to the hearing outlet that sat inside the ear canal, then replace it with a new one each month. Although I have never been a particularly handy person I learnt how to replace the batteries with a reasonable degree of discretion and finesse, but replacing the filters proved to be quite challenging. Somehow, the action of flipping out the old lining and replacing it with a fresh one, an action that seemed effortless in the audiology technician's hands, rapidly became my nemesis. The old one didn't flip out as required and the new one never fitted in as required, resulting in subsequent frequent trips back to the technician who would patiently demonstrate once again the utter simplicity of the procedure.

After paying a fairly astronomic sum for the new technologies in my ears, I now wanted to answer the big question, was I hearing any better? The answer was not that simple and reminded me of the famous curate's egg *Punch* cartoon; the young priest is given a bad egg for his breakfast by the curate and on being asked, "How is your egg?", he replies, "Oh, it's good in parts".

I could hear people next to me better, I could hear a lecturer in a hall better, and I could hear patients in the clinic more clearly. But then there were the other situations. Sitting in a restaurant I was hearing numerous conversations being conducted at adjacent tables, but less from those sitting at my table. At concerts I discovered that I was hearing the rustle of the program pages turning, much more dominantly than the music played on stage. So all in all and despite the explanations regarding the six channels state-of-the-art modern hearing aids, with almost human ability to tune out disturbing tones and focus on the important sounds, the reality was a limited ability to improve my hearing problem. I frequently found myself deciding to leave the aids at home. I preferred adjusting to my known problems while sitting closer to people and watching their lips, than to be bombarded by unwanted sounds impeding my ability to hear normal discourse.

A few years passed and I readjusted to life without hearing aids. I knew I was missing out on conversations and irritating those around me by either ignoring them or requesting that they repeat things. So I finally bowed to reality and returned for another hearing test. The results showed a similar picture and I was persuaded that over the last four years technology had moved on, and it was worth returning to the hearing aids. So now I am fitted out with the newer and better aids which I can adjust for volume, or change the setting so I can hear those closest to me better. I think I am hearing conversations at other tables in restaurants less clearly, and maybe succeeding a little better in holding a conversation with the person next to me. To be completely honest, in a noisy restaurant I will still be doing a lot of polite smiling and head-nodding, hoping that these are occurring at the right time and in the right context.

The seemingly mild nature of my impairment is just another reminder of how much can go wrong in the human body. I manage my daily routine without being conscious of the hearing problem but there are many occasions where I find myself missing the essence of a conversation, or having to ask the person I am speaking with to repeat what he or she were saying. Such behavior contributes significantly to how people perceive me, and hearing impairment makes a significant contribution to the recognition of me as an ageing individual.

As a fairly serious amateur musician, I think that today I appreciate Beethoven more than ever, and certainly see myself as one of his greatest admirers. In his famous Heiligenstadter Testament he describes in great detail the agony of not being able to understand the environment, "...how humiliated I have felt if somebody standing beside me heard the sound of a flute in the distance and I heard nothing, or if someone heard a shepherd sing and again I heard nothing". I am fortunately not there, but often think about the genius of his late quartets or ninth symphony, written when he no longer heard anything. I can only hope that there are enough hair cells in my inner ear or enough technological improvement of hearing aids ahead, to slow my hearing deterioration and allow me to participate in the orchestra of life and normal daily conversation.

About twenty years ago I visited an ophthalmologist colleague and was informed that the time had come to start using reading glasses. My first reaction was feeling hurt and insulted that I was being forced to adopt my first geriatric symbol. On donning the first pair of half lens glasses that rested low on the bridge of the nose, I found some compensatory satisfaction in the new look of the more serious academic paediatrician. The reading glasses were to prove themselves to be an ominous monitor of the ageing process that had begun to kick in.

Visits to the optometrist increased in frequency as the need for stronger reading glasses and then adjustments for other functions steadily increased. There were changes in the ability to see road signs, then adjusting the distance for computer use, and further adjustments required for reading the music while playing string quartets. Finally, the moment of truth arrived when my optometrist suggested I try multifocals. I must confess there seemed to be some logic in this; it became tiring to try and remember which glasses to take to work, to a movie, or when going to play music. Not infrequently, I would find myself with the movie glasses during a Haydn quartet, having to move chairs and adjust lighting to allow continuation of the activity, or going to the movies with my reading glasses. And so, I duly moved on to the next senior moment of ordering multifocals. "It will feel a little strange for the first few days, but then you will adjust to them and wonder why you have waited for so long", reassured me my optometrist as I handed him my credit card to pay a painful sum for the new pair of glasses that included non-scratch, unbreakable lenses which also darkened in sunlight, and basically promised a new view (!) of life.

I marched out of the office to return to work and began to descend the stairs down to the car park. A wave of terror seized me as I suddenly felt like I was standing on the bow of a sailboat in a storm (I feel sick just looking at a sailboat). Luckily, I managed to grab hold of the rail alongside the stairs to stop the imminent fall. I reached my car and managed to drive home but there were many moments of land-based seasickness till I slowly adjusted. Sure enough, I finally learnt the subtleties of multifocals and became attached to them forever. All was well for a few years until the eyes began to deteriorate and adjustments to the lenses were required once again, at increasing frequency.

Nearly a decade following the start of the multifocal era, I returned to my ophthalmologist. Examining me he smiled and said, "Well, there's a small cataract in both eyes. Nothing urgent, but we'll follow them". I dutifully reported for periodic checkups, and then was predictably informed that the said cataracts were growing and it was time to intervene. The thought of any medical intervention to my body was not welcomed at this point of my life. I decided to delay the process by getting second opinions, otherwise known in lay language as "doctor shopping".

I was referred to Dr L, who had done miracles with a colleague's mother. I visited him in his very pleasant consulting rooms with plenty of chairs, television, and a very harassed secretary. I was ushered into his room after a short wait and received a thorough examination of the eyes, followed by a detailed explanation of the problem, demonstrated on a model of the eye. As the indication for surgery was the subjective feeling of the patient, and not the size of the cataract, the decision was mine regarding when to undergo the procedure while assured there was no urgency. This allowed a little more time for procrastinating the surgery, during which I continued the ritual of corridor consultations. The list of names of the miracle workers in the field of cataract surgery expanded, and in addition to the surgeon there was also a list of possibilities regarding the type of lens to be inserted. Modern technology now allowed for a multifocal lens to be inserted theoretically replacing multifocal spectacles.

The final step toward deciding on the surgeon was when I met a surgeon colleague, who described his experience with a certain ophthalmic surgeon working in my health plan. "He doesn't have great interpersonal skills", my surgeon friend remarked, "but the surgery itself took twelve minutes with no after effects". This personal testimonial sounded like what I needed; a good ophthalmic surgeon, working in my health plan, and recommended by a fellow surgeon.

Using some personal and professional connections to reach the said surgeon I received an appointment date, and presented myself for examination. I waited in the busy waiting room (looking more like a train station's waiting room compared to my previous experience), before called in to see Dr K. I pointedly presented myself as Dr Porter, a paediatric colleague who worked in the adjacent building. This was greeted with a terse nod, followed by a few questions, and a review of my previous examinations. I was then examined on two different machines, with minimal conversation, and then reseated opposite Dr K. He duly informed me that there were cataracts, a larger one on the right, and if I was experiencing increasing discomfort now was the time for surgery. I set a date six weeks later which allowed me the time to convince myself that the cataracts were indeed causing me considerable inconvenience, and that it was time for action.

On the appointed day, I worked at my clinic until two pm and then presented myself at the operating rooms for eye surgery. Reading a medical journal in the waiting room until my name was called, I sat pretending to be nonchalant. I was called by the nurse who instructed me to remove all my clothes except underpants, don the hospital gown, and to make sure that the strings to tie the gown were in front.

Once more I was aware of the rapid passage from Herr Doctor Professor to "the next patient". I sat with a ridiculous hospital cap on my head, the gown tied in front allowing many open spaces to view expanses of flesh, and my socks and blue operating room booties to complete the image. Since there was no possibility to read or see television in the pre-surgery and recovery room, staring into space and meditating was the only option for the next half hour or so which felt like eternity.

A young porter approached me with a wheelchair and instructed me to sit in the chair without presenting walking as an option. I dutifully sat in the chair and allowed him to deposit me in the operating room next door, leaving me with a chirpy "Good luck". The operating room nurse instructed me to lie down, followed by the placing of sheets over my face with a hole over the eye due for surgery. Dr K swept into the room and was immediately asked by the nurse why he had not marked the eye for surgery. He quickly reviewed my notes again and then drew a black blot above my right eye. I found this step reassuring. The nurse discovered that a small step in preparation had been missed and reminded the surgeon to check and clearly indicate the eye for surgery.

I thought many years back to my period as an intern when I was working on a surgery unit specializing in vascular surgery. One morning

I was following the young surgical resident as we checked patients after surgery. The elderly gentleman looked up at the resident and asked why the bandages were on his left leg when his pain had been on the right. Without batting an eyelid the resident smiled and said that all was in order. Later, I looked at the notes and saw that the surgery had been performed on the wrong leg. "He'll need it soon on that leg anyway", was the laconic answer. At least things had changed a little in this area over time.

I looked at my watch. Three twenty nine pm. I felt the cool antiseptic liquid cleaning the area around my eye, some drops in the eye, and a muttered "OK" from the surgeon. I then started to see colours and shapes dancing in my field of vision, a slight sensation of pressure on the eyeball, and the sound of a machine. "That's it", said Dr K. The sheets were whisked off and I saw the friendly porter standing next to me with the wheelchair again. I looked at my watch, three forty pm. The whole procedure had taken eleven minutes. I dressed in the recovery room. Dr K reappeared and presented me with the summary of the surgery and a prescription for eye drops. Apart from a little tearing from the eye and a slight gritty sensation I felt completely normal. The follow up visit, the following morning, took less than two minutes. A quick look at the eye was followed by a revision of instructions regarding the eye drops, and then a cheery, "Do the girls look better this morning?"

I had experienced another wonder of modern

medical technology. A procedure that not long ago would have involved a few days of hospitalisation was now performed in the middle of a working day, the entire experience taking two hours. A part in a critical sensory organ had been replaced in a process resembling the assembly line of a car, rather than the mystic glory of human surgery. For the second eye I was better prepared and requested the procedure to be performed when realizing that through the eye with the new lens I saw things in beautiful high density, and clear bright colours, while through the other eye the world looked more like a Turner painting; a little murky-yellow-brown in colour. I returned to the eye surgeon who accepted my decision and a few months later I walked out of his surgery with the second new lens in place.

I cannot say that the difference changed my life. But I could see things more clearly, the colours more vivid. I still needed glasses although I could see things from a distance without them, meaning I occasionally removed my glasses to see things from further away. This meant having to remember that I had removed my glasses and hung them on my shirtfront, before I moved on. Every solution creates a new problem.

The degeneration of the eyes and ears are daily reminders of the ever increasing decompensation of the body as ageing progresses. Glasses need cleaning and another few cells in the memory sections of the brain to remind us where we have left them. Hearing aids need cleaning and battery replacement. Needless to say that the battery usually signals its impending demise, now with a little ding-dong in the ear, at the most inconvenient time and mostly when a replacement battery is not handy. The worn out batteries have come to symbolize for me the other numerous waring out processes going on in my body.

The slowly worsening pain in the knees due to worn out cartilage, the steadily increasing breathlessness while covering the same distance on the regular or irregular walks. And the scariest reminder of the ageing machine, the relentlessly progressive inability to remember names, things, events, and people. Perhaps the brain researchers are getting closer to a memory aid that can connect to the cortex of the brain, hopefully as an inconspicuous chip in the scalp, and send a prodding signal to the appropriate cells and connections as I stand mumbling that I need to contact "You- know-who, what's-his-name, the brother of that other guy, who works in that place".

THE BIG C

And just when I thought that the train wreck and the parotid tumour were my final major body events, the fickle finger of fate struck again.

It was really all my wife's fault. She had been nagging me for a long time to go for a proper checkup, not just a routine visit to talk about pain medication modification. Also, and because I felt I deserved a long break from doctors and hospitals I had not yet done the compulsory colonoscopy test recommended at my age. I reluctantly went to see the doctor, a very professional and experienced family physician. She reviewed my history and lifestyle, and of course suggested I do the routine blood tests and, yes, see a gastroenterologist regarding the colonoscopy.

I decided that I must do it all immediately otherwise I would put it all off, forever. And so, the next morning I had scheduled the consultation with the gastroenterologist, and the following day I was up bright and early to go to the laboratory to do the blood tests. Later that morning I went to see my dermatologist for my yearly check. He stripped me and reviewed my ageing skin including scrotal folds and anal cleft, looking for any suspicious lesion. "All is well", he said, "just a bit of fungal ointment between the toes". It was good to hear that my outer layer was holding up to the ageing process. From the dermatologist I proceeded with my wife to one of Tel-Aviv's finer restaurants to celebrate our wedding anniversary, with good food and a glass of wine, looking out over the beautiful Mediterranean Sea. Returning home, I dreamily lapsed into a delicious nap remembering the asparagus in butter and linguini recently devoured.

The phone rang. "Basil, it's G", said the friendly voice of my doctor sounding a little on the nervous-cum-professional side, "they just called me from the lab… There's a bit of a problem with your tests. The white cell count is 110,000". I paused. *Wasn't this a little high? Quite high? No. It was ridiculously, terrifyingly, deadly high!* "Oh", was the best I could manage trying to think in objective doctor mode. This was not some patient, a relative, or a friend. It was MY body kicking back again. So the salivary gland tumour and the train accident had not closed my account, and a new challenge was now in place.

The first thing I did was to stare at the wall in front of me for a few minutes pondering the rest of my life, while continuing to digest the linguini. My doctor had suggested that I go immediately to the ER at the large medical center near my home. I pictured a young inexperienced internal medicine resident hearing my story, then asking for the haematologist on call to see me, and the three or four hours' wait in the crowded ER full of elderly patients waiting for beds upstairs. This was not a good idea. A moment of inspiration entered my befuddled brain, and I plucked up the energy to call a haematologist friend at a large hospital in Jerusalem. He listened to my description of the latest event, and within five minutes returned with the direct phone number of the senior haematologist at my nearby hospital. Also the haematologist was remarkably quick off the mark, "Can you be here within a half hour?" Shortly after that I left her office with some words ringing in my ears that were partly familiar (Chronic Myelocytic Leukemia, Philadelphia Chromosome), many others that were pretty new to me, and a lot of forms for more blood tests.

If it was CML (Chronic Myelocitic Leukemia), the prognosis was good, due to the state-of-the-art therapy available. I proceeded home to try and carry on with life. "Well there's bad news but also some good news", and, "Yes, it is leukemia, but it's probably the best one to have because of a new set of wonder drugs which offer a full life". These became the mantras of the next few weeks, though I myself was not yet convinced.

Following the results of the blood tests, my haematologist explained that for this disease things would hopefully go well on the single-pill treatment. But first we had to deal with the tumour mass, the enormous number of abnormal white cells being pumped into my bloodstream, which would involve taking some pills by mouth for a week or two. I was certainly happy not to be starting "chemo" - the heavy stuff which was given intravenously and resulted in that attractive bald look, along with vomiting your innards out. At this point my guardian angel haematologist did recommend that I keep away from children for a while. As my immune system might be taking a blow I did not want to catch some infection from the children visiting my clinic, laden with virus and bacteria.

Life now included a new set of routines. A fifteen minute morning walk to the hospital allowed me to collect my thoughts and calm my anxiety level for the experience. I would then enter the hospital and walk the long never-ending corridors before reaching my destination, the Haematology Outpatient Department. I knew enough about managed care to know what to expect next. At the booth, the clerk responsible for authorising the visit and the tests would look at my forms and inform me that I did not have the authorisation for some of the tests that had been ordered. This required going to the office of my HMO at the end of another long corridor, on another floor, with another wait of at least half an hour.

On one of these occasions, just as I was about

to sit down and pretend to read a newspaper, a lady walked out of the office. Seeing me she asked, "Aren't you Dr Porter?" My heart raced and I jumped up as I responded, "Yes, I am". "Oh, I'm Dr Z's daughter." I smiled. My anxiety level dropped. A huge feeling of relief descended. I knew someone. I had the "Magic Vitamin P", protektzia, which is essential for the successful negotiation of any service setting in Israel. I had become a person, not just a number in line. The additional tests were authorised and I went back to the clinic where Rachel, the nurse, proceeded to take the blood specimen. Rachel was a square-shaped lady probably around sixty. Dressed in a green scrub suit she had a constant expression of aggravation on her face. This was not your nurse for compassionate words about your disease, or idle chit-chat about the grandchildren. But she was a supremely efficient blood taker. A task which had now taken on a special significance since most of the juicy veins in my arm had disappeared, due to overuse during my hospitalisation following the train accident.

Strolling back home, via the neighbourhood patisserie for a croissant and latte, it was time to start dealing with the plans, prognosis and wellbeing. Again, the most difficult part as with the parotid tumour and the train accident was the loss of control, and the lack of knowledge as to where this was going, together with the inability to do anything about it. I tried to maintain a daily routine and somehow pretend that all was normal.

Over the following few weeks my white blood cell count began to respond to the medicine, and slowly began the descent to the more normal range. At some point during this treatment my wife decided I needed an outing to take my mind off the disease for a while, and off we went to a museum a pastime I usually enjoy. As we walked through the halls of the Diaspora Museum, embracing the worlds of the Jewish diaspora through the ages, I suddenly began to experience a new sensation of weakness and weariness. This was something new. I had certainly felt tired following the train accident, a post-traumatic exhaustion that persisted for a long time. I had certainly suffered from severe exhaustion after the five-hour surgery to remove the parotid tumour. But this weakness was something alien and frightening. A feeling that I had to be horizontal soon and once down on the bed simply not wishing to raise my head, not to mention the rest of my body.

I returned to Dr N my haematologist and described this new phenomenon of unknown, ongoing, and extreme tiredness. She smiled patiently at me, and proceeded to explain in the simplest layman language that I had been going through a process of removal of the tumour mass. The fact this mass was in my bloodstream, and not appearing as a lump somewhere on my body, it was still a mass - a huge number of ineffective white cells churned out by a machine out of control. I was feeling what any cancer patient feels when their tumour is being hit by chemicals to reduce its size. This was one of many occasions when I realised how weak our vocabulary is when trying to describe symptoms. The weakness during this induction phase of treatment was memorable as a gold standard for defining weakness. It was difficult to describe to my doctor, to my wife, even to myself. It was a feeling of wanting to be left alone, a need to save energy involved in any activity. Be it walking, eating, or talking.

It was also a time to reflect on my energy level in general. I remembered when Dr N asked me how I'd been feeling prior to the discovery of the abnormal white cell count. My answer was quick and straightforward that I had been quite normal, feeling nothing unusual. But now that I was feeling the ultimate exhaustion it seemed easier to see a gradient. Yes, I had been getting more tired than usual. I had found that my walks were getting shorter, considerably shorter. I remembered clearly that up to the previous summer I had been walking for one hour; a pleasant loop down through the park, along the seafront, and back home. Recently, after half an hour I had been turning around and heading home, surprised at my lack of fitness and blaming the rapidity of advancing age. I had been exhausted after a five-hour clinic, feeling a weariness of new proportions, and collapsing on the bed on reaching home. Was I just convincing myself about something that was expected to happen with this illness? The lack of any objective measure of tiredness makes any assessment post facto questionable regarding its reliability.

Over the next two weeks the white cell count slowly dropped back to the normal range. I was ready for the next stage of treatment, the stage of chronic maintenance. I was one of the really fortunate people who when hit by the Big C, had come out of the lottery of life with the first disease to have its genetic defect controlled by a single daily pill. I began taking the magic Gleevec, one pill each morning, together with the pills for my chronic pain. I swallowed them together, pausing to wonder how the white pill knew that it has to go to my brain to block some abnormal pain perception from my spinal injury, while the brown one had to kick in at some bad genes which were producing an abnormal enzyme.

I had also been warned about a long list of potential side effects from Gleevec. It was not the usual explanation given about a medicine using the terminology "possible stomach aches, or rare skin rash". Gleevec seemed to promise deliverance from a bad disease with a heavy price tag attached, both economically and physically. While the economic side was absorbed by the health system, the side effects were a personal price paid by the patient. Whereas with aspirin or a statin the warning would be the possibility of experiencing side effects, here the side effects were presented by my physician as a fact of life. I would experience one, some, or all symptoms which were now well-known after more than ten years of experience with the drug. Swelling of the eyelids or ankles due to accumulation of fluid were the most common things to expect, as well as leg pains, stomach disturbances, or dry mouth. These were mentioned by the doctor.

But when reading the package insert the list increased logarithmically: inability to sleep, dizziness, numbness of the hands, heartburn, flatulence (oh really?), dry eyes, hot flushes, and many more. These were the common side effects. The list of uncommon side effects included anything affecting every organ of the body, and more. To list a few: breast enlargement in men and women, reduced sexual desire, generally feeling unwell, increased urination, and stomach ulcers. The drug insert also had a section listing the frequency of side effects: "Very common side effects *may* affect more than 10 in every 100 patients, common side effects *may* affect between one and ten in every 100 patients, uncommon side effects affected between 1 and 10 in every 1000 patients." How was I supposed to prepare for all this?

I carried on and waited looking in the mirror every morning, to see if my eyes were swollen or reddened, and checking my ankles for edema fluid. And just as I was starting to feel that once again the side effects issue was being overdone, to ensure legal coverage for the drug company, I began to notice some gnawing pains in my calves. The pains were not severe, just bad enough to cause discomfort and a little feeling generally unwell. Fortunately, the pains responded well to simple pain remedies and enabled me to carry on my normal routine. And then, upon convincing myself regarding my superior ability to defy the package inserts for the drugs, a new surprise awaited me.

I awoke one morning, walked to the bathroom, stripped for my shower, and saw strange new phenomena covering my body. Huge red spots covered my legs and torso, my skin was as dry as sandpaper, together with various degrees of itching. I raced back to my doctor who directed me to the dermatology clinic. After a considerable wait a pleasant young doctor reviewed my notes, looked briefly at my body, and declared that this was a classic acute eczematous eruption (I already knew that…). He then proceeded to enter the issue of eczema and CML into the Internet, finding of course that this had been reported. Just like the drug insert said. He then patiently explained to me the required regime to manage the problem including twice-daily baths with a soothing oily medium, an oily cream to be applied afterwards, and cortisone cream to follow. To my delight after a few days of delicious soothing baths, and following the regime of creams the rash rapidly disappeared. My skin, at least in some parts, was now smooth and almost reminiscent of the proverbial baby's bottom.

I returned to Doctor N. She pondered with me whether in view of the allergic reaction there was a need to try the second-line drug that had entered the market. It seemed that the Gleevec miracle was followed by the discovery of additional drugs which were also taken by mouth, and recommended to patients experiencing severe reactions to Gleevec. We decided on a period of "watchful expectancy" before making the change. I have always liked this well-worn metaphor of medical care. The idea of a period of watching before jumping to change a treatment and the "expectancy" indicating that while watching we would be ready to expect change, a good pillar of medical care.

This decision also indicated another reason for my adulation of Dr N. She related to all decisions as a process of consensus. True, part of this was due to her seeing me as a colleague. But I had no doubt that this was how she practiced her art, and over time I had the opportunity to witness her in action with patients in the day hospital. She always approached the patient while sitting on a movable stool which enabled her to sit opposite with direct eye contact. She always opened her contact with, "How are you feeling today?" or some variation thereof. Then she actually listened to what the patient said even if he or she rambled, or lectured, or just complained. She always had time, and always listened before saying her piece. She always gave the patient the feeling that the decisions were shared ones. She knew the importance of helping the patient feel in control. And even if in the end decisions were professional and could only be made by her, with her extensive knowledge, the patient always felt he or she were part of the process.

I was really no different from any other patient, just lucky to have a treatable disease with relatively little suffering involved. Still, each time I left my meetings with her I felt empowered and in control of my problem. Even if she had been delayed in coming to see me because of a serious problem, arriving two hours later than expected, after our ten minute meeting I would walk out smiling. This was the art of medicine in practice, a combination of superior knowledge and skills with the ability to listen and talk straight to the patient. During my waits in the day hospital, I had plenty of time to ponder the burden of an empathetic academic physician, managing a caseload of patients most with severe life-threatening disease, who always had time for everyone. She understood that despite the advances in medicine, the wondrous new drugs, and the ability to reach the basic cause of many diseases, still the basis of good medical care was the doctor-patient relationship.

As I write, I am celebrating four years of treatment of my CML. I am in complete haematologic remission, and monitoring my disease. This includes routine measuring of the abnormal gene fractions responsible for the disease which are showing better than expected response, and I also feel in excellent health. Every morning, swallowing the large brown pill, I consider myself blessed. Although I could officially categorise myself as one of the Living with Cancer group, I had been spared the reality that most cancer patients face; the severe pain, the wasting away, and the confrontation with one's mortality. I am able to see myself as one of the normal people, able to keep up a normal routine and reflect on mortality from the viewpoint of anyone approaching the eighth decade, without cancer prognosis being at the forefront of my thinking. I also reflect on the fact that if I had been diagnosed with CML only fifteen years ago, the prognosis for the disease would have been poor. I would have had to experience intensive and exhausting chemotherapy, spending most of my days in a day hospital setting, would have experienced multiple hospitalisations, and the chances of being alive after five years would have been slim.

The increasing understanding of the genetics of cancer is showing that at the root of all cancer is a genetic glitch. I was fortunate to be hit by the first cancer that the genetic defect was identified and the specific treatment so fine-tuned that it seems one can indeed talk of cure. Clearly, the path to curing all cancer will ultimately depend on exhaustive research into the genetics of each type of cancer, occurring in patients with a variety of genetic makeups, with a long pathway still ahead.

A while ago, I went to my nearby hospital to have my blood tested for the molecular monitoring of my disease. Although four years had passed since the fateful day when I had been diagnosed with CML, the hospital still caused an anxiety reaction. As I reached the security check at the gate I already felt the familiar sweating in the armpits and the racing of my heartbeat. At least I knew the routine which was now down to every three months, as opposed to daily or weekly in the early stages. I was more confident that there would be no major surprises in the results, and I also knew the ropes of the hospital bureaucracy.

It was two minutes to eight am when I reached the reception desk of the haematology clinic that was just opening. "First in line today", I flashed my most charming smile at the familiar clerk, and pushed my authorisation form from my HMO through the gap in the window. Careful not to make any eye contact she put on her usual scowl, and perused the form. I watched as her eyes squinted slightly before she pushed the form back to me. "This is the wrong code number for the test", she declared, perhaps with a slight note of triumph in her voice. "You'll have to get a new authorisation from the senior haematologist at your HMO". I paused, pondering whether to start making a scene, declaring my status as someone with the right contacts, a doctor and professor, or maybe drop the name of the hospital director. But then I quickly realised that the hatchet-face at the window was used to these scenarios, and probably thrived on them.

I trudged down the endless corridor to the HMO office in the hospital, and saw that the reception windows were all closed. Without hesitating I opened the door used by the staff, and saw a single familiar face sitting opposite a computer screen. She looked up with an expression of rage ready for the fight. "Hello S", I smiled, "how are you? And how's your dad?" She stared at me for a moment before breaking into a smile of welcome. I was a known person, not another nuisance in the line.

I explained my problem, adding that I had a clinic in another half hour and had to do things as quickly as possible. She perused the form and explained that she had to get authorisation from another secretary, and was not sure whether I might have to resubmit my request for authorisation. She suggested that I take a seat while she tried to take care of this as soon as possible. Forty minutes later she exited from her cubicle, proudly handing me the new authorisation. I thanked her profusely, sent regards to her father, and dashed back to the haematology clinic. My secretary in my clinic had already called to say that the first patient was waiting.

I reached the haematology clinic and to my relief no one was waiting for blood withdrawal. I entered the room and found one technician explaining to a colleague a learning module on the computer. I raised myself to full height, breathed deeply, and explained once more that I was a busy paediatrician and children were already lined up in my clinic. "Just a minute", I was told, and they proceeded with their task. After a further few coughs and shuffles one of them grudgingly rose and attended to me. She strapped my arm and barked at me to open and close my fist. I explained that it was difficult to find veins in certain places, but was shushed away. Sure enough, she slipped the needle under the skin and I immediately knew she had missed the vein. She put on a face of stern confidence and declared that she had been in the vein just the blood did not flow. The other arm was strapped.

I watched as she quickly attacked the other arm where veins were usually found, but in my case were rare in this arm after previous repeated traumas during hospitalisations. I was about to get up and declare that I would come back next week. Then, to my surprise and delight, the thin line of blood appeared in the tube attached to the needle. My blood letter triumphantly drew the sample into the tube and attached the necessary labels. "At least this confrontation with the system had ended successfully", I mumbled to myself as I dashed off to my waiting patients and their mothers in my clinic.

I had been spared the miseries of most cancer patients; the repeated hospital visits for chemotherapy causing vomiting, loss of appetite, exhaustion, depression and more. I am spared the uncertainty regarding my prognosis not knowing whether the treatment will cure me, prolong my life, or have no effect. The wonders of one-pill-a-day therapy have enabled me to experience the aggravation caused by a clerk, regarding a bureaucratic authorisation for a test, as the major trauma in the management of my disease. True, I am a doctor and I know people. Following my diagnosis of CML within an hour I had not only found a top specialist to manage my disease, but that same person presented herself as being my future Medical Home. She gave me her office, home, and mobile phone numbers as well as her email. She had essentially declared that she was my address for all concerns, and directed her secretaries and nurses to ensure that I would not have to endure the bureaucracy more than minimally necessary. I could also call the director of the hospital, a previous close colleague of mine, and bring forward a complicated imaging procedure for a friend with a progressive malignant disease.

Having experienced my boutique care I am highly aware how crucial the process of care is to the wellbeing of the patient, and how rarely this process is managed appropriately. My thoughts often wander to the masses of patients out there who do not have the cash or connections to achieve what is needed in the quickest and least bureaucratic way. And also how easy it is to lose all proportion. How quickly one forgets the terror of the initial uncertainty accompanying the cancer diagnosis, and how quickly banal issues of everyday life easily replace the fear of losing life itself.

SO WHAT DOES THIS ALL MEAN?

At this point hopefully I have managed to convey my message. Mainly that there are a lot of bad things that can happen to one's body, and that a combination of luck and advances in medicine seem to have allowed me to enter my eighth decade functioning relatively well. Some people may define luck in more religious terms, but I have seen too many religious people, from the mildly to ultra-orthodox, being struck by all the bad things while prayer and penitence did not seem to have effected their outcome. I am sure this is a simplistic view, but I still find it easier to involve just Lady Luck, with apologies if there is indeed a higher source guiding my destiny.

Also, I do not claim to be unique with my experiences even among my closest circle of friends. One friend had his prostate gland removed after a raised PSA[15] level in a screening test suggested early cancer. This test has recently been the subject of multiple articles in the medical press. Some claiming it allows for detection and removal of cancer at the earliest stage, while other studies have shown that many people with these very early cancers live out their lives and die of other causes, not prostate cancer. The luckier event for this same friend was finding a malignant melanoma of the skin at the earliest stage, enabling treatment and full cure. If it had been discovered six months or a year later, it would have probably advanced to a stage where cure was unlikely.

Another close friend had a melanoma diagnosed and treated early. But before declaring cure, his final follow-up CT of the whole body showed an incidental finding; a widening of a portion of the aorta - the large artery exiting the heart, which indicated an early aneurism - a weakening of the wall of the blood vessel that could have burst at any time and invariably be fatal. Successful surgery for removal of the affected area of the aorta followed, and he is back to normal function at work and home.

---

15. Prostate Specific Antigen - the higher the man's level of PSA the more likely he has prostate cancer

Stories of this kind lead one to reflect on how it all works. Some people will go for any new report on a vitamin or food supplement which has been shown to prolong life, strengthen the immune system, prevent heart disease, or even improve sexual function. I have been impressed that women seem to have a greater belief in these measures to save or prolong life, watching some of them swallow large quantities of colourful pills with their meals. Most of the men I know may swallow a statin and an aspirin to ward off heart attacks, but will be less likely to stalk the health food stores and pharmacies seeking the panaceas to longevity and good health. Another aspect is lifestyle. There is no question that younger and older, fat and thin, female and male, sick and well, have all caught on to the importance of lifestyle. The two most evident parts of it center on exercise and nutrition. Namely, that sensible eating and moderate exercise are good for your health, will improve the quality of your life, and will probably enable you to live longer.

Reflecting on the things described in the preceding chapters none seem to have been preventable, at least regarding knowledge available at the time. True, if I had been a little more alert on Hampstead Heath I may have been able to avoid the car approaching at slow speed before contact was made. But almost all the other events were dependent on medical interventions.

Today, few patients with appendicitis will reach an advanced stage of the disease without the problem being identified by a simple ultrasound.

Few adolescents have to suffer their acne for long before being treated with the new drugs targeting the basic problem, without disfiguring the skin. My severe jaundice and subsequent gallbladder disease probably all date back to a genetic defect affecting the management of bile pigments, together with an infection caused by the Hepatitis A virus. Today the virus can be controlled by a series of vaccines given in early infancy with a later booster, so even mild jaundice is relatively rare these days. My three major life events: the tumour of the salivary gland, the train accident and the leukemia, at first glance do not seem preventable. Could the salivary gland tumour have been connected to Dr L's radiation of my face for acne some six decades earlier? The only answer to that is, maybe. Radiation certainly is associated with later cancer. But whether the low radiation delivered and the benign tumour years later indicate cause and effect? This is definitely no more than a guess. In view of my train accident, should one recommend only sitting in the middle carriages facing the back to prevent being derailed and flung about in the event of an accident? Was my leukemia a fluke genetic mutation, or connected to radiation from a medical source or the environment?

I think back on my maladies, the yearly recurring sinusitis syndrome that sometimes paralyzed my functioning for weeks, not to mention those who had to listen to my orchestra of coughing and spitting, while trying to remove secretions from my sinuses. The unremitting itching during hepatitis, that gave me some suicidal thoughts, and a simple word like

Colic that took on new meaning when I personally experienced my gallbladder trying to pass small stones down the tube linking to the bowels. The waves of increasing pain reaching a crescendo of agony, when only a loud scream could offer some relief. There is no doubt that the center player in the symptom catalogue is certainly pain.

Reflecting back on my life health issues, pain is the central symptom for describing suffering. Pain brings the curtain down on the stage of normal living, distorting thinking, emotions, and everyday functioning. When I met the word pair *Neuropathic pain* following my train accident, a new avenue of suffering opened up, different from all the other pains experienced in my life. The realisation that pain could be there all the time varying in intensity or quality, but always there, was an idea not present in my overview of life as a doctor or a patient. Like parrying with a regular opponent on the sport field, learning the vagaries and trying to build strategies to meet the challenge, it took a good five years for me to be able to understand this new adversary.

Dealing with a new chronic pain was also part of a journey of coping, a process of learning the intricacies of a problem challenging my health, then moving on to a strategic plan to manage the problem within the context of one's life routines. All these personal experiences with disease and trauma relating to my body changed my attitude as a doctor, more than any lecture in medical school or clinical experience. I think I was always a fairly empathetic doctor, someone who could listen to a patient talking about their problems while conveying a caring and understanding demeanour. But each experience as a patient added a new layer of understanding to the true meaning of empathy.

Not being able to remember today what I had for dinner yesterday, I can retrieve each incident in my life relating to inadequately empathetic physicians and nurses. I remember the frozen features of the famous surgeon deciding he needed to explore what was happening in my abdomen at age twelve, compared with the cheerful smile of the anaesthetist reassuring me before putting me to sleep. I remember lying for hours staring at the ceiling in the tiny sluice room alone and fearful before undergoing gallbladder surgery. The impatience of the nurse examining me in the emergency room after having been knocked over by a car, her main reaction relating to the problem of finding a cubicle to put me in, with no understanding of my level of pain and dizziness. And the cherry on the top, the plastic surgeon examining the pressure sore on my scalp, following a nearly fatal accident, who did not even bother to relate to me as a human being under his care.

Much of my desire to describe my personal history of disease stems from a feeling of frustration with the way doctors related to me, not to me as a doctor, but to me as a patient. I was taught, as all future doctors are, that the patient history is crucial to diagnosis. Many students and teachers in medical schools today see technology as the solution for pinpointing all ills. An ultrasound or CT will be ordered for a complaint such as stomach aches, headaches, or chest pain, without worrying about a good history taking. History taking, as I was taught in a first-rate medical school, was an inventory of questions. A basic checklist aimed at getting facts about the presenting problem, and a review of all other systems of the body. So through the history we would start with stomach pain, then proceed to how long, how intense and the type of pain, whether at a specific point or more diffuse, and whether it comes and goes. This was important information which could frequently already provide a strong clue as to whether we were dealing with a mild tummy ache, a serious case of appendicitis, or maybe something else altogether.

Today, medicine is more complicated than just performing a series of Sherlock Holmes type activities and deductions, until closing in on the culprit. Medicine today frequently involves people with many complaints related to many systems, and problems that become chronic and don't go away. To understand these kinds of problems we have to get to know more about the people themselves, their lifestyle, their work, their families, and their stories.

Realising the complexity of chronic problems the traditional history has been replaced by the concept of the narrative, i.e. that every patient has a story to tell and if the doctor fails to understand the patient's story the management of the problem will be incomplete. When I presented myself to a gastroenterologist because of my recurring bouts of pain in my abdomen, I was thinking of my father's history of recurrent ulcers in his duodenum, and was convinced that this was where I was heading. But fortunately the specialist delved more carefully into my narrative, and suggested that the problem may be in the gallbladder. Or the trauma surgeon who took my hand, listened to my complaints, reviewed all my imaging and tests, and explained to me that I had experienced multiple trauma not just trauma to my spine with a broken vertebra in the neck.

Medicine today requires curiosity and a readiness to listen, without the restraints of time or a checklist. For those willing to listen to the doctor who had been in a train accident there were messages of pain, physical discomfort, and concern about the future. The social worker chatted with me about my work and family, and a psychologist encouraged me to talk about my feelings. But I needed to hear words of encouragement and reassurance from a physician. It would not need to be more than "This chronic pain is frustrating, but we'll get on top of it", or "Hang in there", while sitting at eye level with me. Only after many years in medicine and some of the bad experiences I have described, did I really begin to understand the importance of quality time - the few minutes that a doctor could devote to listening, smiling, explaining and reassuring, or at least displaying some empathy and an understanding of what the patient was experiencing.

Much of the doctor-patient relationship is dehumanizing; becoming another number in the stream of humanity sitting in a crowded waiting room, or hospital emergency room looking for the medical system to cure real or imagined illnesses. Then, donning the hospital pyjamas and lying in a hospital bed are additional steps in the removal of all previous distinguishing characteristics of the patient. The judge, the street sweeper, and the physician all become "the patient in bed number four".

So then the big question is: can we teach empathy? From my experience as a doctor, academic, manager, teacher, and patient, it seems that it is not an all or nothing issue. Nobody is born a fully empathetic doctor, and anyone involved in treating people can learn elements of empathetic behavior. I think the plastic surgeon who tore the bandage off my pressure sore on my scalp is not necessarily a wife-beater or sociopath. I would guess he is a highly self-opinionated character, who believes he knows best about everything related to his field of medicine. Surely, there were many opportunities during his training to modify his behavior. Also, if he saw his department head greeting every patient with a smile and "How are you?", as a consistent model of how things should be done on a routine ward round, he would probably not have behaved with me as he did. I'm not sure he is a character I would socialise with, but his basic doctor-patient behavior pattern is modifiable.

As I think back to my role models relating to

communication with patients, some dating back to the clinical ward rounds in medical school, a large number were surgeons. I still have vivid memories of one of the high society surgeons, who taught us in the public hospital, who would routinely take the hand of the patient before asking how he or she felt. That small act settled into my memory as the right way to do things. On a surgery ward round with a prominent surgeon, I remember him carefully questioning an elderly gentleman regarding his bleeding from his rectum. When had the bleeding started, was it painful, and then he asked what colour was the blood, a question which could indicate if the blood came from high up in the alimentary tract, or from the rectal area. The patient fixed the surgeon with a stare and asked, "So they make it in different colours now?" At this point all of us together with the surgeon collapsed laughing.

Then there were some of my mentors during residency training. Some paediatric surgeons would effortlessly change the diaper of a baby, while others the moment they saw or smelled the soiled diaper called on the nurse for help. Remembering how much I had been impressed by my mentor who would perform this basic task, during my subsequent paediatric career, I always changed diapers myself. My haematologist, who sat on a low stool and conducted a conversation with every patient while looking into their eyes, displayed a combination of readiness to listen, patience, and understanding. Even the surgeon in Boston, who removed the tumour in my salivary gland, left his mark by explaining exactly what he would be doing; the details of the surgery, how long it would take, and what was I to expect afterwards, his description reassuring and thankfully correct. Unfortunately, I only saw him briefly following the surgery, before he disappeared to a surgical meeting and left me with some disappointment that I did not have another opportunity to ask questions.

All these vignettes helped cement in my mind that communication was an essential part of healing. In the world of modern medicine with the abundance of technology and high pressure workloads on medical staff it sometimes seems that the doctor-patient relationship is dead or dying. The excuse given frequently is lack of time and that the need to be continuously doing specific activities; taking a medical history and examining the patient, contacting specialists for consultation and reviewing laboratory results, all preclude the possibility of spending time listening to the patient. But showing empathy is not necessarily time-consuming. A cheery greeting while establishing eye contact with the patient in bed or sitting across the desk are a declaration of readiness to be the doctor who can help, whether the problem be the flu or major surgery for cancer. Any addition to the smile and eye contact is value added. And a joke about the hospital food, the weather, or the political situation will help cement a bond, a critical part of the healing process.

Today, few days pass without a friend, family

member, or acquaintance relaying a story of poor experience with the health system. The milder complaints will focus on the lack of continuity in care, the lack of a patient manager, or the difficulty accessing certain doctors in high demand. The more significant complaints invariably relate to experiences in hospital emergency rooms or wards, particularly with elderly parents. Ninety-year-old patients often spend days lying on a trolley in a corner of the emergency room while waiting for a bed on the wards, or lying in a corridor next to the kitchen or nurses station. These stories seem more the norm than the exception. They have become the ultimate humiliation for the patient feeling isolated and an irritation to ward staff, rather than an elderly frail person in need of sympathy and a kind word.

I recall my arrival in the rehabilitation unit from the surgical ward following my spinal injury. It was an early Thursday afternoon and the ward was a picture of commotion. Preparing to wind down for the weekend respite, nurses were running around, patients and families clamouring to sign out for the weekend, and the call buttons next to the patients' beds were ringing in a cacophony of bell sounds. A nurse approached me, glared at the papers in my wife's hand, and shouted, "Why do they transfer patients at this time?" Declaring categorically that Dr Porter was not welcome. How different would this have been, "Hello there, sorry things are a bit chaotic on Thursdays at this time. Please be patient while we organise your bed". I would have smiled, relaxed and felt good about my new home. How long would this interchange have taken? Maybe thirty seconds? I will never forget the smile of the woman serving the meals in the rehabilitation ward who saw me coming and would say, "Hello, your favorite schnitzel today". I smiled, we connected, and she had helped me get through another day.

It is hardly surprising therefore that most of the bad experiences with hospitals boil down to the lack of communication frustrating patients and their families. Sadly, the only way to mobilise communication in the system I know is to mobilise protektzia (connections). Namely, finding someone who can persuade the staff that you or your family member are somebody, a person, a friend of Dr X, a relative of the ward chief, etc. Suddenly, the same nurse or doctor who previously did not establish eye contact or exchange a sentence with you now return with a smile and some conversation, "Oh, you know Prof Y?" And a bond has been created. Now you are somebody, a person they actually see. Now you can approach the doctor or nurse, ask a question, and receive a civil answer.

My saga of seven decades of experiencing "interesting" medical and surgical issues as patient and doctor is over. Surely, there will be additional events leading to the ultimate cardiorespiratory arrest. I have lived through an amazing period of advances in medical science. Surgery and anaesthesia, together with understanding genetics and the use of targeted drugs for treating genetic defects in cancer, have enabled me to reach my present age. I stand poised at the end-stage of the human lifespan pondering the future as most do at this age. It is a big game of chance and luck now, with the main hope being that the end will still take a few years, and even more important that it will be swift and painless. I also hope that the doctors I meet along the way, besides being competent and updated in their field know how to smile and say, "Hi, how are you feeling today?"

EPILOGUE

I look in the mirror and see a fading grey hairline. The eyes are a little droopy looking, the upper lids creeping over the line of vision, indicating a possible need for eyelid uplift to keep my vision unobscured or maybe just for vanity's sake. Two new lenses inside my eyeballs following cataract surgery are not visible, but the world looks more colourful and focused since their placement. If one looks carefully, a thin tube of plastic is visible just behind the ears connected with a small plastic capsule holding computerised information behind each ear. The tubes and computers, only partly successful, aimed at trying to retrieve the hearing lost due to damage to the ear passage many years ago. The face also shows some small dimpled scars, particularly in the grooves next to the nose. A zigzagging scar starts at the middle of the lower lip and proceeds down beneath the chin, and up towards the left ear. Another thin white scar is visible under the chin on the right side. It carries on down the length of the neck covering the area of the third vertebra replaced by a man-made copy. And at the back of the neck is a strip of titanium nailed along the length of the neck vertebrae. The abdomen shows two dramatic lengths of scar tissue: one proceeding from the right of the belly button down towards the groin area, the other lying like a centipede under the diaphragm - the roof of the abdomen. Over the right side of the right knee two small spots of scar tissue indicate the insertion of the arthroscope - the machine allowing a view inside the knee joint. The skin of much of my body is now covered in a myriad of coloured spots some darker than others including numerous patches of dry, dead skin, no longer readily replaced as in earlier years. The delinquent gene which has resulted in uncontrolled production of white cells, now controlled by a single tablet taken each morning, has left no external sign.

A body more than seven decades since creation is showing the wear and tear of normal ageing, together with the signs of the ongoing fight against adversity; whether from within via ill-behaved genes, infectious processes, or from outside sources of modern day trauma such as a poorly focused car driver, or a mismanaged train ride. Amazing advances in surgical technology and drug research have helped this body, and many others, to keep up with daily life that so far had been worth the fight. Still, we all know that the most fantastic robots and computers, the most skilled technicians, and the most experienced doctors, will not be able to keep the finger in the dyke forever.